Using Polyvagal Theory to Optimize Healthcare Excellence

Using Polyvagal Theory to Optimize Healthcare Excellence

Randy Brazie
NeuroConsulting Group LLC

Geoffrey Vanderpal
NeuroConsulting Group LLC and Purdue Global

Abi Blakeslee
NeuroConsulting Group LLC and Somatic Experiencing International

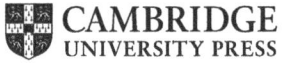

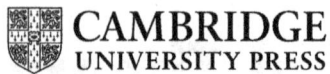
CAMBRIDGE
UNIVERSITY PRESS

Shaftesbury Road, Cambridge CB2 8EA, United Kingdom

One Liberty Plaza, 20th Floor, New York, NY 10006, USA

477 Williamstown Road, Port Melbourne, VIC 3207, Australia

314–321, 3rd Floor, Plot 3, Splendor Forum, Jasola District Centre, New Delhi – 110025, India

Cambridge University Press is part of Cambridge University Press & Assessment, a department of the University of Cambridge.

We share the University's mission to contribute to society through the pursuit of education, learning and research at the highest international levels of excellence.

www.cambridge.org
Information on this title: www.cambridge.org/9781009675932

DOI: 10.1017/9781009675949

© Randy Brazie, Geoffrey Vanderpal, and Abi Blakeslee 2026

This publication is in copyright. Subject to statutory exception and to the provisions of relevant collective licensing agreements, no reproduction of any part may take place without the written permission of Cambridge University Press & Assessment.

When citing this work, please include a reference to the DOI 10.1017/9781009675949

First published 2026

Cover image: Science Photo Library / Getty Images

A catalogue record for this publication is available from the British Library

A Cataloging-in-Publication data record for this book is available from the Library of Congress

ISBN 978-1-009-67593-2 Paperback

Cambridge University Press & Assessment has no responsibility for the persistence or accuracy of URLs for external or third-party internet websites referred to in this publication and does not guarantee that any content on such websites is, or will remain, accurate or appropriate.

For EU product safety concerns, contact us at Calle de José Abascal, 56, 1°, 28003 Madrid, Spain, or email eugpsr@cambridge.org

---

Every effort has been made in preparing this book to provide accurate and up-to-date information that is in accord with accepted standards and practice at the time of publication. Although case histories are drawn from actual cases, every effort has been made to disguise the identities of the individuals involved. Nevertheless, the authors, editors, and publishers can make no warranties that the information contained herein is totally free from error, not least because clinical standards are constantly changing through research and regulation. The authors, editors, and publishers therefore disclaim all liability for direct or consequential damages resulting from the use of material contained in this book. Readers are strongly advised to pay careful attention to information provided by the manufacturer of any drugs or equipment that they plan to use.

Contents

About the Authors vi

Introduction 1

1 **The Polyvagal Theory 101** 4
  What Is the PVT? 4
  Origins of the PVT and the Science of Safety 6
  Core Concepts of the PVT 8
  Potential Contributions of the PVT to Healthcare 16
  Polyvagal-Informed Exercises to Explore and Regulate ANS Function 17

2 **Developing ANS-Focused Clinical Interventions** 30
  Integrating the PVT in Healthcare 30
  Steps for Implementing Polyvagal-Informed Interventions in the Healthcare Setting 32
  Combining the Concepts in the Healthcare Setting 53

3 **Polyvagal-Informed HRM Policies and Procedures** 60
  The Impact of Bias and Discrimination on Recruitment and Selection 61
  Polyvagal-Informed HRM Practices for Mitigating Bias and Discrimination 65

4 **Leadership and Management in Healthcare** 75
  Stress and Trauma in the Healthcare Setting 76
  Practical Leadership Styles for the Healthcare Environment 78
  Leading Workers in High-Stress Healthcare Environments 79
  Embracing Steadfast Leadership 88
  Common Characteristics of Good Leaders 90
  Polyvagal-Informed Strategies for Leading in High-Stress Environments 91

5 **Measuring Outcomes to Improve Healthcare Success** 98
  Challenges in Assessing PVT Intervention Outcomes 99
  Measures for Assessing Mind–Body Outcomes 100

6 **Designing Healthcare Environments That Promote Well-Being** 109
  The Impact of Environmental Factors on the Sense of Safety 110
  The Importance of Appealing Design 111
  The Importance of Conducive Workplace Layouts 113

7 **Interfacing with External Stakeholders** 118
  External Stakeholder Management 119
  Marketing Polyvagal-Informed Interventions 122

Conclusion 125

References 126
Index 132

About the Authors

Dr. Abi Blakeslee is an expert in the field of trauma recovery and the founder of Implicit Psychotherapy. She is senior faculty at Somatic Experiencing International and legacy faculty for Dr. Peter Levine's Ergos Institute for Somatic Education. She is Director of Training and Education at the NeuroConsulting Group. Dr. Blakeslee holds a PhD in clinical and somatic psychology and an MA in counseling and depth psychology. Her dissertation generated original research on the role of implicit memory in healing trauma. Dr. Blakeslee integrates the study of implicit memory and psychophysiology in clinical research, secondary trauma interventions, neuroconsulting, and the psychobiological principles of attachment and shock trauma. She treats individuals, couples, children, and families in her clinical practice. Dr. Blakeslee teaches and consults worldwide.

Dr. Randy Brazie is a graduate of the University of Arizona College of Medicine (1994) and completed his psychiatry residency at the University of Arizona Affiliated Hospitals in June 1998. He has been board certified by the American Board of Psychiatry and Neurology in general psychiatry since January 2000. Dr. Brazie has extensive experience working across multiple sectors, including both clinic and hospital-based services, as well as in emergency and urgent care settings. He also has been active in leadership roles across multiple organizations, in both the United States and New Zealand. He currently serves as a medical director for Blue Cross and Blue Shield of Arizona, as well as running a small private practice and teaching for various universities and colleges intermittently. He has coauthored *The Steadfast Leader* (2023, McGraw Hill) and several professional journal articles with Dr. Vanderpal. He is the cofounder of NeuroConsulting Group, LLC.

An experienced professor and a former financial advisor, **Dr. Geoffrey Vanderpal** is a Certified Financial Planner™ and Chartered Life Underwriter with years of industry experience and has taught for various universities on four continents in the areas of finance and business. Dr. Vanderpal is published in multiple research journals and authored a book titled *Invincible Investing*. Dr. Vanderpal is currently a professor in the Master of Science in Finance (MSF) program at Purdue University Global, teaching financial planning courses. He is the coauthor of *The Steadfast Leader* (2023, McGraw Hill) and cofounder of the NeuroConsulting Group, LLC.

Introduction

The pursuit of wellness often feels like an elusive quest. The uncharted territories of the human mind and the intricate web of the autonomic nervous system (ANS), specifically the function of the vagus nerve, have left many healthcare professionals grappling in the dark. Some seek answers to improve their patients' health and well-being, while others seek knowledge to strengthen their proficiency in delivering care to patients. This book is relevant to both types of seeker.

Using Polyvagal Theory to Optimize Healthcare Excellence aims to impress upon healthcare professionals the necessity of applying the polyvagal theory (PVT) to their practice to positively affect the autonomic states of the individuals they encounter as well as their own. The journey begins with an in-depth exploration of the fundamentals of the PVT in clinical settings and then gradually narrows down the implications of the theory's application in human resource management and leadership.

It is well-known that healthcare professionals experience a high degree of stress and burnout. What's more, rising costs and regulatory burdens negatively impact recruitment efforts and the retention of qualified individuals. This has resulted in an unprecedented shortage of healthcare workers. The healthcare industry cannot continue down this path if we hope to have quality, affordable healthcare well into the future. But change only begins in an organization when leaders recognize the need to shift focus and implement practical approaches. It also begins with individuals taking leadership of themselves by better understanding how the human body responds to stimuli and knowing how to shift out of an undesired state.

In our groundbreaking book *The Steadfast Leader* (McGraw Hill, 2023), we (Brazie and Vanderpal) set out to teach leaders how to stay focused and make good decisions amidst the myriad challenges and opportunities they face virtually every day. With our extensive experience in business, healthcare administration, and healthcare delivery, it made perfect sense to make the leap from general PVT-focused leadership to PVT-focused leadership specifically in the healthcare industry; thus, this book came to be. We requested that Abi Blakeslee, SEP, CMT, MFT, PhD, come on board with us to share her valuable insight into the healthcare industry. As Director of Training and Education for the NeuroConsulting Group, LLC, Abi provides expertise in incorporating concepts from neuroscience, psychology, and related healing professions into practical and powerful knowledge.

Using Polyvagal Theory to Optimize Healthcare Excellence is based on our combined research, unique and shared experiences, and our passion for sharing the knowledge and ideas surrounding the PVT and its application. Chapter 1 ventures into the heart of the PVT, revealing its profound implications for healthcare organizations. The PVT fundamentally reimagines our approach to the ANS by ushering in an era where the three states of

ANS function – *the ventral vagal, sympathetic,* and *dorsal vagal* – are considered allies for promoting our overall well-being. The polyvagal ladder is a visual roadmap to these states, showing how we can ascend the ladder through innovative interventions, offering patients and healthcare professionals the power to self-regulate and shift toward the ideal ANS state of safety and social engagement. Applying the theory can contribute significantly to increased productivity, reduced stress, and the alleviation of burnout, ultimately fostering a healthier and more supportive society.

Chapter 2 shifts focus to the practical applications of the PVT in healthcare. Understanding the cues of safety has become paramount for ensuring that healthcare professionals and their patients feel safe in their respective environments. Historically, healthcare has been rooted in cognitive psychology, which focuses on the workings of the mind, but the PVT's holistic approach reshapes our understanding, urging us to also consider the state of the body. As we delve into evidence-based clinical measures and techniques, the transformative potential of the PVT becomes increasingly evident. This chapter equips healthcare practitioners with essential polyvagal-informed strategies to use and teach to staff and patients. Additionally, this chapter explores somatic (body-centered) psychology interventions and group dynamics that can collectively empower everyone on the journey toward health and well-being.

Chapter 3 examines the multifaceted impact of stress and trauma on the recruitment and selection process in healthcare settings. It explores various influences affecting critical human resource management activities, such as recruitment and selection. Through the eyes of leadership at Safe Haven Medical Clinic, we uncover the effect of stress and trauma on talent acquisition, both implicitly and explicitly. The chapter narrows down the sources of implicit and explicit bias that usually manifest during the talent acquisition process. Furthermore, it provides several polyvagal-informed strategies that modern healthcare professionals should use to create a workplace that thrives and promotes fairness for all employees.

Chapter 4 turns to the topic of leadership in high-stress healthcare environments. Given that the healthcare sector is often associated with work-related stress and trauma, this chapter revisits Safe Haven Medical Clinic as the leadership struggles to navigate a crisis. Building off that scenario, the focus moves to four leadership styles, each of which displays a different aspect of the PVT: transactional, transformational, situational, and servant leadership. Following an exploration of the strengths and weaknesses of each leadership style is an analysis of several polyvagal-informed strategies that leaders in the healthcare industry can employ to improve employees' well-being and overall decision-making. In our previous book, we introduced our concept of "instinctive leadership" to describe the model of a PVT-informed leadership approach. We realized, however, that *instinctive* wasn't quite descriptive enough. Therefore, in this book we chose the term *steadfast leadership* to highlight the interplay of cognition and more primitive brain circuitry in leadership behavior.

Chapter 5 introduces practical methods for assessing the outcomes of polyvagal-informed strategies. Despite the emergence of various approaches to measuring the outcomes of different psychology interventions, there are still significant obstacles when assessing the efficacy of polyvagal-informed approaches. To rectify these issues, this chapter recommends several approaches for assessing the outcomes of polyvagal-informed interventions, placing the focus on four types of measures: (1) objective measures, (2) behavioral observation, (3) subjective reports, and (4) standardized psychological assessments.

Healthcare leaders can compare the strengths and weaknesses of these measures to determine which offers the best assessment.

While previous chapters focus on PVT concepts and the influence of internal sensations on decision-making, Chapter 6 moves the focus toward external sensations. Factors such as building designs, lighting, audition, and olfaction can play a vital role in conveying safety to patients, healthcare workers, support staff, and leadership. Accordingly, this chapter expounds on the relationship between the environment and cues of safety to create the foundation to highlight how conducive building designs and workplace layouts can improve employees' mood and well-being. The ultimate objective is to create an environment that communicates safety to those within it.

Chapter 7 revolves around external stakeholder management. Healthcare delivery is a continuum that involves the participation of both internal and external stakeholders. While internal stakeholders, such as healthcare workers and leadership, took priority in the earlier chapters, it is crucial to understand the role external stakeholders play in the delivery of polyvagal-informed practices. As such, this final chapter highlights how healthcare facilities can inform payors, providers, media outlets, and learning institutions of the benefits of implementing polyvagal-informed strategies and interventions in healthcare settings. What's more, this chapter describes the most efficient practices for marketing a polyvagal-centered program and presenting the evidence-based findings of these interventions.

Join us on this journey as we unlock the riddle of the autonomic nervous system to understand how polyvagal-informed strategies can shape various elements in today's healthcare sector. As we journey further into this book, we'll delve into the practical applications and groundbreaking interventions informed by the PVT and describe their implementation to solve real-life healthcare scenarios. Welcome to the world of healthcare built on the principles of the PVT – a world where the human nervous system paves the way toward optimal health and healing.

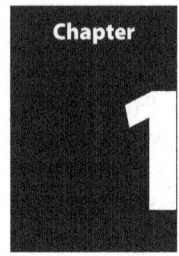

Chapter 1

The Polyvagal Theory 101

While the term "polyvagal theory" (PVT) may sound lofty and academic, it is quite straightforward and applicable to the real world once you know the basics. In this chapter we discuss the origins and key concepts of the PVT. In addition, we describe the effectiveness of conceptual models, such as the polyvagal ladder, which are used as guideposts to map changes in a person's autonomic state. This chapter also highlights the potential contributions of the PVT to the healthcare sector and healthcare professionals. This chapter closes with several polyvagal-informed exercises, which you can start using immediately: first with yourself to experience the effects firsthand, and ultimately with staff, colleagues, and patients. We'll also visit the Safe Haven Medical Clinic in this chapter to illustrate these concepts.

Objectives
- To define and explain the origins of the PVT and its relevance to mental health and well-being.
- To explore the core components of the autonomic nervous system (ANS) and their function.
- To apply the model of the polyvagal ladder to the three states of the ANS and acknowledge how and why this can be a positive contribution in healthcare.
- To become aware of neuroception and interoception, the methods by which we monitor the external and internal environment for signs of safety or danger.

What Is the PVT?

The PVT is a groundbreaking paradigm that connects the neurological mechanisms responsible for generating feelings of safety with social interactions and overall well-being. Developed by Dr. Stephen Porges and introduced in 1994, the theory offers a profound understanding of how human beings' physiological responses and emotional states are entwined with their ability to connect and thrive in social contexts. From Porges's perspective, the theory proposes that "social connectedness is tantamount to stating that our body feels safe in proximity with another" (Porges 2022).

The theory proposes that the ANS, which includes the parasympathetic nervous system and the sympathetic nervous system, has three distinct physiological and behavioral states: the ventral vagal state, the sympathetic state, and the dorsal vagal state. These states are associated with different functions and responses. For instance, the ventral vagal state is linked to social engagement, safety, and relaxation; it determines a person's ability to connect with others. In comparison, the sympathetic state is associated with the fight-or-flight response by preparing the body for action when it perceives a threat. Last, the dorsal vagal state is responsible for immobilizing the body when it detects an extreme or constant threat (the freeze state). Both the ventral vagal state and the dorsal vagal state are parasympathetic responses, but with significant differences. The shift between these three states is the cornerstone of the PVT; as such, we will be examining these three states throughout the book.

Although contemporary science emphasizes the importance of understanding a person's biological needs, it is quite common for people to ignore the influence of their feelings and physiological states on their biological functions. In reality, a person's sense of safety is closely tied to their physiological state, which is regulated by their ANS (Porges 2022). The polyvagal perspective underscores that feelings of safety serve as the fundamental underpinning for comprehending human social interactions and behaviors. By emphasizing the ANS as the central player in determining whether an individual perceives safety or threat, it becomes possible to predict their inclination toward the fight-or-flight response. In simpler terms, when someone is in a calm physiological state, this state tends to promote social engagement, fostering positive interactions and prosocial behaviors. Conversely, when someone is in a tense physiological state, this state tends to lead to defensive action or avoidance behaviors.

Therefore, the polyvagal perspective highlights the critical role of feelings of safety as a foundational aspect of human anatomy and physiology. On this note, "a polyvagal perspective clarifies the evolutionary transition that enabled mammals to be social and to use sociality as a mechanism to regulate and optimize physiological state and homeostatic processes" (Porges 2021a, 1). Porges explains that the evolutionary advantage of being human lies in humanity's ability to evolve into social mammals. He emphasizes that a human being's capacity to form social connections can be attributed to their internal systems and their ability to maintain a state of balance within their nervous system.

Again, the polyvagal perspective takes into account the three main states of the ANS described in the PVT: the ventral vagal state, the sympathetic state, and the dorsal vagal state. Each of these states is associated with specific physiological responses and behavioral tendencies, and they can be dynamically activated in response to environmental cues and perceived safety or threat. Therefore, the underlying basis of the polyvagal perspective lies in its inherent focus on perceiving the ANS as a uniform system comprised of multiple branches that have evolved to perform specific functions.

Taking these ideas into consideration, the PVT is a key concept in the science of safety. The ANS can be compared to an internal barometer that determines when a person has been subjected to an impending threat or too much stress. Trauma, anxiety, and stress can play significant roles in stimulating the ANS to shift from the ventral vagal state to the sympathetic state or the dorsal vagal state. Normally, when all is well we stay in the ventral vagal state of social engagement. When our nervous system detects cues of potential danger, we transition either to the sympathetic state of mobilization or the dorsal vagal state of immobilization.

Polyvagal-informed interventions is a term that reflects the idea of creating environments that exude safety for target individuals. Awareness and understanding of polyvagal-informed practices, policies, and environments can promote healing and strengthen resilience against stress. However, polyvagal-informed interventions are not quick fixes to mental health problems; rather, they are step-by-step approaches for improving physical, mental, and emotional well-being.

The Relevance of the PVT in Healthcare

Dr. Stacy Jennings has a PsyD in behavioral health and currently works as the chief clinical officer of Safe Haven Clinic, a general outpatient clinic. The facility provides a wide variety of mental health services to patients on an outpatient basis. Her specialization in behavioral health provides her with a strong understanding of various mental health issues affecting society.

Dr. Jennings has always been a keen observer. Her discerning eye has helped countless patients navigate the labyrinth of their mental health challenges. However, something troubling has caught her attention in recent months. Over the last eight months, the clinic has recorded a gradual uptick in the number of patients grappling with fear, stress, and anxiety.

Among the struggling patients is 45-year-old Fred Johnson, who has social anxiety disorder. A once-energetic man, Fred has become a virtual recluse. Even the simplest interactions trigger severe anxiety and stress. Fred is at his best when he feels safe and connected. He usually finds solace in the company of a few close friends who understand his condition. However, when he is invited to a large social gathering, he usually becomes tense, his heart starts racing, and his palms become sweaty. His body is preparing for a fight-or-flight response driven by his fear of social interaction. As his anxiety intensifies, Fred becomes physically and emotionally overwhelmed. His voice quivers, and he often freezes when speaking. In such cases, he prefers to withdraw to a quieter space where he feels safe.

Recognizing the urgency of the situation, evidenced by all the distraught faces in the waiting room, Dr. Jennings gathers her team for a routine meeting. The PVT was the main topic of discussion: Whilst attending a conference focused on trauma and anxiety treatment research, she had been introduced to the PVT and was impressed by its scientific basis and outcomes.

The clinic's conference room, typically a place of clinical discussions, became an arena of intellectual exploration. With passion, Dr. Jennings shared the theory's origins, tracing it back to the pioneering work of Dr. Stephen Porges. She explained that the PVT is more than just a theory – it is a key to understanding the ANS and day-to-day social interactions. Dr. Jennings painted a vivid picture of the PVT's core components, using Fred Johnson's case as the foundation.

We'll revisit this scenario and Fred's case later (see "Helping Fred Up the Ladder"). For now, the relevance here is that Dr. Jennings was equipped with the information she needed to start creating change where she clearly noted change was needed.

Origins of the PVT and the Science of Safety

The PVT derives most of its concepts from historical research on the functions of the ANS. Before the 1900s, researchers conceptualized the ANS based on the responses of the vagus nerve. The vagus nerve is the tenth cranial nerve, which originates in the brain and connects to a wide variety of body organs, including the facial and eye muscles, the heart, the lungs, and the intestines. Incidentally, *vagus* means "wanderer," reflecting how extensively the nerve travels through the human body.

The founding fathers of the PVT are Charles Darwin, John Hughlings Jackson, Paul MacLean, and Stephen Porges (Hays 2019). Foremost, in the 1870s Charles Darwin proposed that emotional expression is reciprocally linked to a person's physiology through the vagus nerve. From his perspective, the vagus nerve bidirectionally exchanges information between major organs of the body, particularly the heart, lungs, and abdomen.

Following Darwin's theory, in the 1880s John Hughlings Jackson proposed that the nervous system operates in a hierarchal manner whereby the higher nervous system controls or inhibits the lower nervous system. This explains why some people are suddenly rendered functionless in extreme situations. While Darwin's theory clarified the mind–body connection, Jackson's theory highlighted the dynamic hierarchical relationship in the body. In 1966, Paul MacLean offered a comprehensive description of the phylogenetic development of animals, particularly reptiles, mammals, and human beings (Hays 2019). Maclean's clinical and laboratory investigations discovered significant evidence that coincided with Jackson's ideas. These three researchers provided considerable insights that were incorporated into Dr. Porges's research when he conceptualized the PVT.

In the early to mid 1900s, research in psychophysiology and psychosomatic medicine largely revolved around the simplistic idea of antagonism between the parasympathetic and sympathetic nervous systems. Accordingly, many researchers had a limited understanding of crucial concepts such as autonomic balance, sympathetic arousal, and vagal tone because they did not possess a deep understanding of the specific neural pathways and feedback mechanisms involved in regulating the ANS (Porges 2021a, 1). At that time, the understanding of the vagus nerve in mammals primarily focused on its role as an undifferentiated motor pathway that regulated various organs, without giving due consideration to its sensory feedback loop. However, Dr. Porges altered the direction of research by highlighting the unique traits of the vagus nerve in human beings and the role evolution plays in allowing the body to respond to environmental changes. Porges's model offers a more complete description of how a human being's body makes unconscious decisions, especially when exposed to stress and other types of pressure (Hays 2019). Over the years, the PVT has become a reliable model for explaining neuroanatomical and neurophysiological processes in animals and human beings.

Based on Porges's hypotheses, the PVT unveils the intricate neural mechanisms behind mammalian social engagement, survival, and communication. As a result, it sheds light on how cues of safety and threat impact a person's ANS and well-being. Instead of focusing on human beings' similarities with ancient vertebrates, it concentrates on the adaptations that set mammals apart to optimize their survival. The theory emphasizes the transition from reptiles to mammals by highlighting the neural adaptations that enabled human beings' cues of safety to influence their state of defense or nondefense (Porges 2022, 2).

Central to this theory is the concept of a uniquely mammalian social engagement system. This social engagement system comes to life in the relationship between mothers and their nursing offspring. For survival, mammalian infants must nurse efficiently, a process dependent on the ventral vagal pathway. As these offspring mature and socialize, this circuit becomes the neural platform for sociality and coregulation (i.e., the supportive process between two people that fosters self-regulation) (Porges 2022, 2). The circuit also supports essential homeostatic functions aligned with health, growth, and restoration. Accordingly, turning off unwarranted threat reactions shifts the nervous system from a state of defense, allowing the ventral vagal pathway to activate and strengthen social connections and a person's sense of calmness. Based on this rationale, Porges categorized the ANS as an intervening variable that mediates human reactions in response to fear or other extreme emotional states.

In response to these insights, the PVT emerged to transform psychophysiology from a descriptive science, merely documenting correlations between psychological and physiological processes, into a solid concept for understanding the relationship between mind and body. It aimed to generate and test hypotheses related to common neural pathways governing both mental and physiological processes. This theory marked a pivotal shift in the field of cardiovascular psychophysiology by challenging conventional knowledge and creating more opportunities to increase society's understanding of the intricate mind–body interplay.

Core Concepts of the PVT

The PVT describes how our nervous system constantly scans both the external and internal environments for any sign of danger or problems. These signs could be real or perceived. If potential danger is detected, the vagus nerve is involved in trying to protect the organism by turning on or off a state of defense. We know this as either a fight-or-flight response or dissociation in the case of severe stress from which we cannot escape (to try to survive the danger). When no danger is perceived, the system then allows a state of relaxed social engagement to come online.

Major Divisions of the ANS

The ANS is a critical component of the nervous system that controls various involuntary bodily functions, such as heart rate, digestion, respiratory rate, and other critical functions. Two major divisions of the ANS are the sympathetic nervous system (SNS) and the parasympathetic nervous system (PNS). Two components of the PNS are the dorsal vagal complex (DVC) and the ventral vagal complex (VVC). The DVC, VVC, and SNS are interconnected and run parallel to one another. Let's consider the location and function of each.

- The DVC, located in the medulla oblongata of the brainstem, regulates a portion of the parasympathetic branch of the ANS. It represents an evolutionarily older component of the ANS found in all vertebrates (Winter and Tyree 2021). One of its main functions is to regulate and connect the brain with organs such as the stomach, intestines, and heart. When this pathway is activated, it tends to slow down the heart and conserve metabolic resources. The DVC is associated with the dorsal vagal state, usually referred to as immobilization (or "freeze").
- The VVC includes brainstem regions and the ventral motor nucleus of the vagus nerve. It is considered a newer evolutionary system that is most prominent in mammals (Winter and Tyree 2021). The VVC is responsible for connecting the brain with organs such as the lungs, esophagus, vocal muscles, and facial muscles. It forms a connection with the "vagal brake," a node in the heart that is responsible for keeping the heartbeat steady and regulated to effectively meet the needs of the moment and to "put the brake on" during activity when an immediate reaction is needed that does not require a full SNS response. The VVC is the primary pathway that is active when we feel safe and able to connect socially with others. It is the most advanced part of the mammalian nervous system.
- While the SNS originates in the spinal cord, it is interconnected with and communicates with various regions of the brain, including the hypothalamus, which plays a central role

in regulating autonomic functions and coordinating the body's response to stressors (Porges 2011). The primary function of the SNS is to prepare the body for immediate action in response to perceived threats or stressors by activating a wide range of physiological responses to help the body cope with challenges. Thus, this pathway is associated with the flight-or-fight response.

Understanding how our nervous system is organized and functions around safety and danger allows us to better grasp how and why we react to stress and real or perceived risk. In many cases, being exposed to stress and/or trauma tends to cause the nervous system to "pull the alarm" and determine there is a threat, even in the absence of one, as an anticipatory protective mechanism. The brain prefers to call a false alarm and survive, rather than potentially miss a real alarm and not survive! In learning about how we are hardwired and respond in various situations, we can then begin to think about ways to help support the nervous system to return to a state of calm, safety, and connection when appropriate, and help to retrain it away from a tendency to assume danger when it is not present.

Figure 1.1 illustrates the central nervous system to help you visualize its structure and connections. You can see that the brain connects to the spinal cord, and from there sends many connections to every part of the body, largely to control motor functions and gather sensory input (letting us know how things are going in all systems).

Figure 1.2 is a simplified illustration of the social engagement system of the ANS. This figure illustrates how the brain connects via the cranial nerves to the muscles of the head and neck. These muscles control how we communicate and connect with the external world – for example, alerting others when we are friendly, angry, or fearful. These cranial nerves also impact our heart and respiration, helping us to prepare for fight-or-flight (mobilization) or energy conservation (immobilization) when a threat is detected. This connection is bidirectional, such that a person's social interaction can influence their psychological state and vice versa.

Based on the PVT, the evaluation of risk does not require conscious awareness, as human beings have an unconscious automated process of threat detection, defined by Porges as "neuroception" (there's more on this in the following section). Overall, the PVT highlights the ANS as a central structure for responding to signals of safety or threat from one's internal system (body organs) and external surroundings (immediate environment). In other words, much of how we respond to people and circumstances is handled by the body without our conscious awareness. From the baseline of evolutionary biology, we are simply predesigned to react and respond.

Neuroception and Interoception

The PVT highlights the relevance of neuroception and interoception in understanding how our physiological responses are intricately linked to our emotional and behavioral states.

Neuroception describes the reflexive process by which the ANS detects cues of safety or threat in the environment. As we've established, this is a neural process that operates beneath conscious awareness and is responsible for evaluating environmental and visceral cues as safe, dangerous, or life-threatening (Porges 2021a, 5). This mechanism is not limited to humans. Neuroception is similar to nociception (the reaction to pain) in that it triggers rapid responses to threats even before the source is identified or consciously perceived.

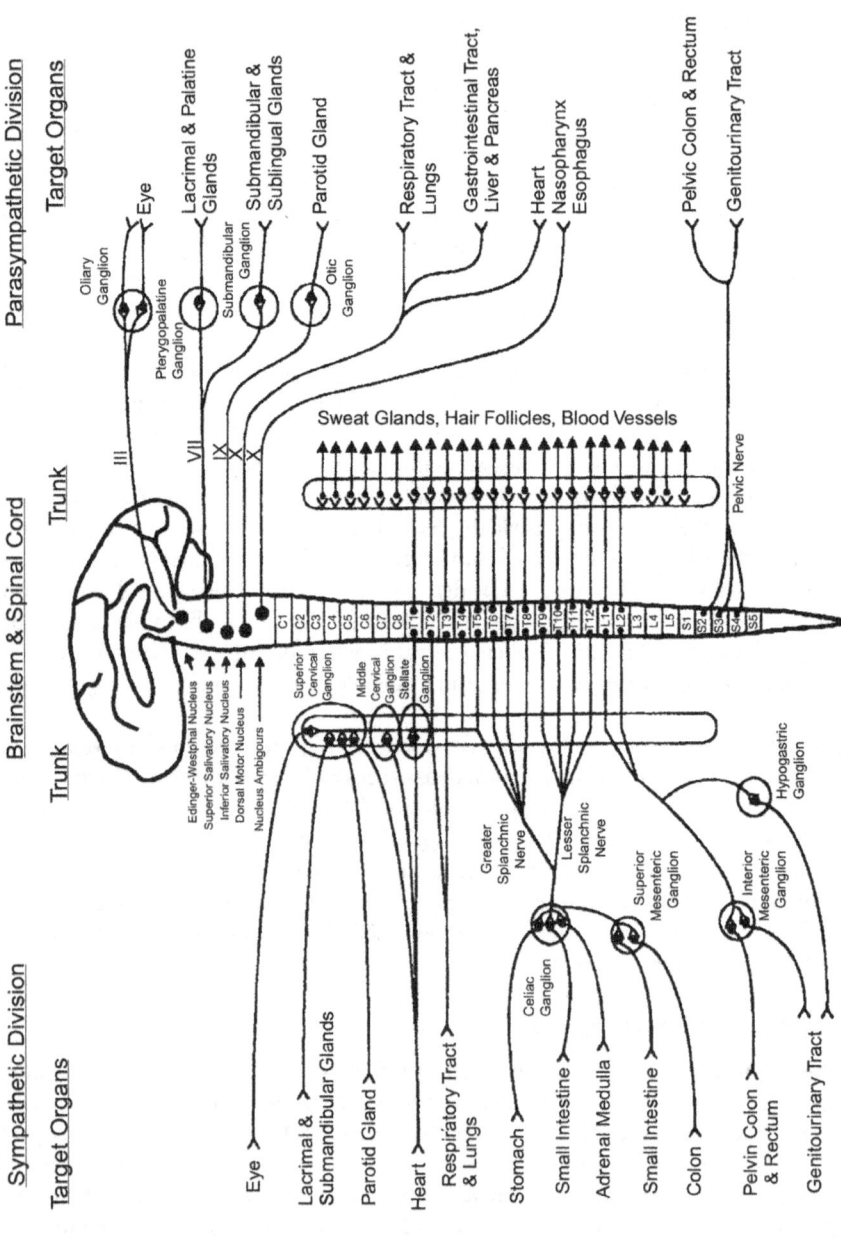

Figure 1.1 Schematic diagram of the sympathetic and parasympathetic divisions of the ANS. (Source: Hamill et al. 2012, 18.)

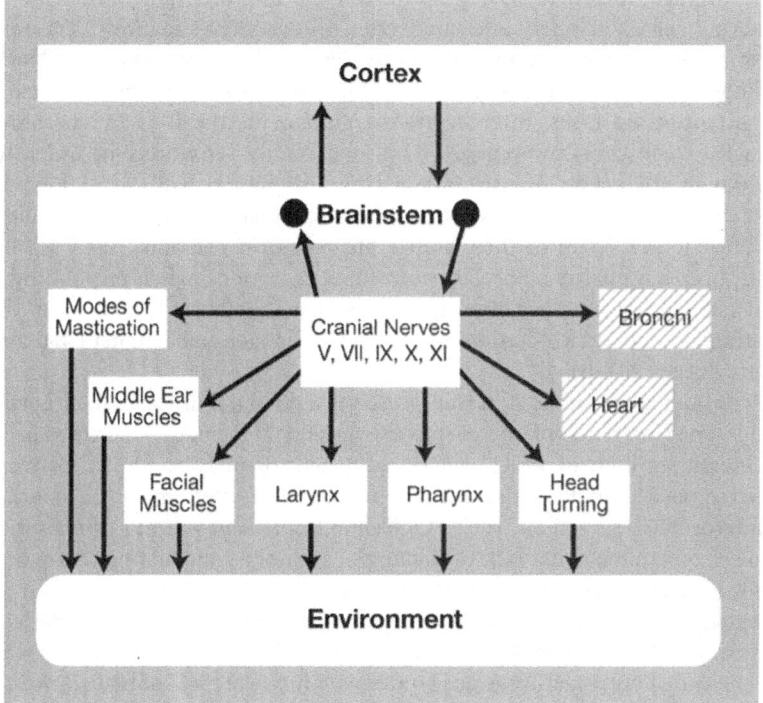

Figure 1.2 Social engagement system. (Source: Porges and Kolacz 2021.)

In humans and other mammals, neuroception goes beyond mere threat detection; it enables immediate responses to cues of safety as well, facilitating the downregulation of defensive strategies. This downregulation promotes sociality, allowing for psychological and physical proximity without the risk of injury. This calming mechanism adapts autonomic function by reducing sympathetic activation. Neuroception decodes the presumed goals of biological movements, such as facial expressions, gestures, and sounds, enabling the nervous system to respond to the intention behind them, sometimes resulting in positive social interactions.

On the other hand, we have *interoception*. This term first appeared in scientific journals in the early 1940s; however, similar terms such as "interoceptors" and "interoceptive reflex" were used prior to this in Sherrington's 1906 book, *The Integrative Action of the Nervous System*. Dr. Bud Craig defined the term "interoception" as pertaining to the role of the insular cortex (a distinct lobe of the cerebral cortex) in bridging conscious awareness with bodily sensation. This refers to a person's *conscious* awareness of their internal bodily signals based on processes such as heart rate, breathing, digestion, and emotional states. In essence, interoception can be considered the sixth primary sense that serves to support the external senses (vision, audition, touch, smell, and taste) (Porges 2011). This is a direct way to "read" your polyvagal state, allowing you to regulate your ANS as needed.

With polyvagal-informed strategies, we can use interoception to increase and promote internal senses of safety and connection in everyday situations. The increase in a sense of safety and connection leads to greater well-being, a more confident sense of self, feelings of satisfaction, better relationships, increased performance, and sustainment of attention on tasks. Interoception complements the PVT by emphasizing the importance of conscious awareness of internal bodily sensations in order for us to monitor our internal state to ensure we are functioning normally, as well as to provide clues as to when neuroception has detected cues of danger. As a result, individuals often become consciously aware of their body's physiological reactions, such as changes in heart rate, breathing patterns, or gastrointestinal sensations, when responding to safety or threat cues. These interoceptive signals provide valuable information to the brain, contributing to the interpretation of safety or danger and influencing autonomic responses (Porges 2021b).

Let's consider an example: A person perceives a potential threat in their environment. Their heightened awareness of interoceptive signals might include an increased heart rate or shallow breathing, both of which can signal a fight-or-flight response. Conversely, the person perceives a friendly environment. Their sense of safety might be associated with calmer interoceptive sensations, such as a feeling of pleasant warmth or relaxation in the body, slower breathing, and a lack of shaking or tremors, contributing to a more relaxed autonomic state and social engagement behaviors.

Understanding and enhancing interoception can help people become more aware of their physiological states, potentially aiding in emotional regulation and stress management through the use of polyvagal-informed strategies. This awareness of body process is called *embodied cognition*. In her 2014 book, *Sensation: The New Science of Physical Intelligence*, Thalma Lobel writes

> Embodied cognition theory proposes that the mind cannot work separately from the physical world; that the senses provide the bridge to both our unconscious and our conscious thought processes. We psychologists and neuroscientists working in this field seek to show the influence that physical sensations have over our mental states and behavior. The mind–body connection is evident in everything we do. (Lobel 2014, 12)

Interoception, as a concept, is a foundational aspect of mindfulness-based approaches. The tendency under states of stress is to ignore our own sensation and instead focus on trying to identify and mitigate sources of potential danger. Thus, we benefit from reconnecting with our inner sensory experiences, as this tends to help break the cycle of being fixated on and distracted by stress. See the "Neuroception and Interoception Practice" section for relevant exercises.

The Three States of ANS Function

Now that we have introduced the basic concepts of PVT, let's dive into the three states of safety versus danger that the nervous system moves between. The polyvagal ladder was created by Deb Dana as a way to visualize this. We invite you to bear with some repetition, as this discussion will help reinforce what you have learned so far. To recap, we move between a state of socialization, where we determine we are safe and can connect with others, to a state of mobilization, when we may need to confront or evade perceived danger, and finally to a state of immobilization, where our neuroception decides that we cannot avoid danger.

- **Ventral Vagal State (Socialization):** The ventral vagal state (or socialization state) describes the capacity of the ANS to engage in positive social interactions and form connections with others when one is in a safe environment. In this state, the ANS fosters calm behavioral states, allowing people to effectively engage in social communication. Being in this state helps inhibit the SNS's influence if a fight-or-flight response is not warranted by actual danger. When the ventral vagal state is active, people have an increased sense of satisfaction and equanimity when alone or with others and display friendly and approachable facial expressions, vocalization, and increased active listening, thereby allowing them to create connections with others (Porges 2007). Therefore, the ventral vagal state is the state wherein socialization and positive social behavior thrive. This leads to increased satisfaction in the workplace as well as in one's private life.
- **Sympathetic State (Mobilization):** The sympathetic state (or mobilization) is characterized by the activation of the SNS to trigger the fight-or-flight response, particularly when one is exposed to an impending threat/danger or is facing a challenging situation. When the SNS is dominant, physiological responses such as increased heart rate, heightened alertness, and muscle tension occur to prepare the body for action (Porges 2007). The sympathetic state is essential for stimulating one's survival instincts in the face of immediate danger, and it also plays an important role in helping us to meet challenges, complete tasks, and even enjoy a sense of play.
- **Dorsal Vagal State (Immobilization):** The dorsal vagal state (or immobilization) occurs when a threat is perceived as too overwhelming, leading to the physiological shutdown of the body. The dorsal vagal state represents the most primitive component of the ANS. In this state, the individual may experience a physiological shutdown of their body, which can manifest as behaviors such as feigning death, fainting (vasovagal syncope), and behavioral shutdown (e.g., emotional detachment or apathy, loss of motivation or social withdrawal) (Porges 2007). The dorsal vagal state is a last resort in response to extreme threats. Shared with most vertebrates, it represents a state of physiological and behavioral shutdown aimed at conserving energy and reducing the risk of further harm.

What Is the Polyvagal Ladder?

The polyvagal ladder (or autonomic ladder) is a conceptual framework that illustrates the hierarchical relationship between these three distinct states. This theory likens these states to ascending rungs on a metaphorical ladder. According to Dana, each state is accompanied by unique physiological, emotional, daily living, and health attributes. With this additional information, the polyvagal ladder is an effective tool for categorizing the factors that cause a person to shift from one autonomic state to another.
- **Top Rung of the Ladder: Socialization State** – The top of the polyvagal ladder signifies that an individual is at the optimal social engagement levels. In this state, individuals experience feelings of safety, connection, and positive social interactions. From a physiological perspective, the heart rate maintains an effective equilibrium. In addition, breathing becomes deep and unhurried, facilitating an enhanced capacity for oxygen intake and promoting a sense of tranquility. The individual's sensory perception is also heightened, allowing them to effectively engage in social activities. With regard to

emotions, individuals residing in the social engagement system often experience a harmonious blend of positive emotions. As a result, these individuals are usually inclined toward prosocial behaviors and are usually willing to form connections with others (Dana 2018). The health benefits of this state include regulated blood pressure, a healthy heart, a strong immune system, quality sleep, good digestion, and a general sense of vitality (Dana 2018).

- **Middle Rung of the Ladder: Mobilization State** – When an individual descends from the top of the ladder, they enter the mobilization state. Physiologically, the heart rate escalates, increasing the delivery of oxygen and nutrients to meet the demands of heightened alertness in accordance with the fight-or-flight response. The person begins to breathe shallowly and rapidly to optimize oxygen intake for peak readiness. Metabolic resources are redirected toward immediate action, thereby strengthening one's physical capabilities for confrontation or escape. However, this state tends to result in daily challenges and health complications when the person is in mobilization for extended periods. For instance, individuals who spend an inordinate amount of time in the mobilization state usually grapple with a spectrum of intense emotions, such as anxiety-related conditions, concentration issues, and strained interpersonal relationships (Dana 2018). Furthermore, health complications such as high blood pressure, heart disease, weight gain, sleep disturbances, memory issues, and various stress-related conditions may manifest (Dana 2018).

- **Bottom Rung of the Ladder: Immobilization State** – The immobilization state is activated when an individual perceives overwhelming threats that leave them feeling trapped and helpless, rendering them incapable of the fight-or-flight response. Physiologically, the immobilization state results in the shutdown of bodily functions. This response includes a reduction in heart rate, often to levels significantly below baseline. As a result, blood pressure may drop precipitously, contributing to the feeling of lightheadedness. The immobilization state is a survival mechanism that allows the body to conserve resources when all options seem futile. With regard to emotions, an individual in the immobilization state struggles with despair, abandonment, and disconnection from the external world (Dana 2018). Accordingly, for someone who is in this state for an inordinate amount of time, daily life can become quite challenging because the individual may struggle with memory issues, dissociation, extreme isolation, depression, and pervasive fatigue. In addition, various health consequences can manifest, such as chronic fatigue, gastrointestinal disturbances, persistent low blood pressure, type 2 diabetes, and weight gain (Dana 2018). These physiological and emotional burdens underscore the role of the immobilization state as a last-resort response to overwhelming adversity.

Figure 1.3 illustrates how Dana represents the polyvagal ladder visually, with the ventral state at the top and the dorsal vagal state at the bottom. The individual using the ladder template is invited to think about how they experience each of these three states by describing how "The world is … " when in that state and what they notice in themselves ("I am … "). Empty boxes to the right at each level invite the person to label that particular state with their own word(s), if desired.

Figure 1.3 The polyvagal ladder. This visual representation of the three ANS states (ventral vagal, sympathetic, and dorsal vagal) invites the individual to think about how they perceive the external world and themselves when in each. (Source: Dana 2018.)

Helping Fred Up the Ladder

As Dr. Jennings described it to her staff, Fred thrives when he is in an environment that exudes safety and connection, particularly when surrounded by close friends who empathize with his social anxiety. This optimal state at the top of the polyvagal ladder manifests as a stable heart rate, deep and unhurried breathing, heightened sensory perception, and an overarching sense of peace. Emotionally, positivity propels him toward prosocial behaviors and the establishment of meaningful connections with others. The associated health benefits are manifold, encompassing regulated blood pressure, a healthy heart, a robust immune system, quality sleep, efficient digestion, and an overall sense of vitality.

However, Fred's mobilization is triggered by circumstances that exacerbate his social anxiety, notably large social gatherings. In the middle of the ladder, his physiological responses are marked by a faster heart rate, shallow and rapid breathing to optimize oxygen intake for heightened alertness, and the redirection of metabolic resources for immediate action. Emotionally, this state is characterized by the emergence of anxiety-related conditions, concentration issues, and strained interpersonal relationships. As a result, daily challenges arise whenever Fred grapples with the fight-or-flight response. This leads to his avoiding social situations due to his overwhelming sense of fear and an urge to flee.

Fred feels immobilized when his sense of neuroception determines that he's either in danger or in a stressful situation from which there is no escape. Fred's response in the immobilization state is characterized by a heightened state of emotional and physiological distress triggered by severe social anxiety. His breathing becomes more constricted, and his overall bodily functions enter a state of conservation and self-preservation. As the immobilization state is linked to feelings of powerlessness and a sense of being overwhelmed, Fred's anxiety has reached a peak, leading to a state of mental and emotional paralysis. For that reason, he struggles to engage with others and finds it difficult to express himself verbally. He may even experience a state of dissociation. This state encourages him to withdraw into a self-protective shell as a coping mechanism.

Dr. Jennings needs to consider appropriate polyvagal-informed strategies to support Fred's ascent back up the polyvagal ladder. Additionally, she can use these techniques to incorporate cues of safety in the waiting room, helping all the patients feel more at ease. As the staff starts to understand the potential positive effects of applying the PVT to healthcare, their excitement grows and they are eager to learn more about how to reduce stress and burnout and find more enjoyment in their jobs.

Potential Contributions of the PVT to Healthcare

Historically, researchers relied on inefficient approaches to understand the neural mechanisms behind cognitive and physiological processes. At that time, the inadequacy of healthcare technology limited scientists' ability to understand the neural mechanisms behind the nervous system. As the scientific approaches to neuroanatomy and neurophysiology expand, more interest has been dedicated to the impact of neural structures on social behaviors and mental health issues such as depression, posttraumatic stress disorder, and autism (Porges 2003).

Currently, however, the rapid advancement of modern medical practices, such as imaging techniques, has provided researchers with a reliable strategy for analyzing brain function and structure in living beings. With these breakthroughs in technology, new opportunities have emerged for investigating the neurophysiological correlations and influences of the human body's major organs. The continuous advancement of this field of research has gained significant attention in the healthcare sector due to the growing need to improve the health and well-being of modern patients and those who care for them.

The PVT offers a reliable framework for understanding somatic psychology, a field of psychology that focuses on the relationship between the mind and the body. Conventionally, assessing safety requires one to search for the presence or absence of threats in one's environment. While this approach has merit, it does tend to oversimplify the concept of safety, neglecting its intricate connection with human social behavior and well-being (Porges 2015). This gap poses a major hindrance to contemporary healthcare professionals who seek to apply the PVT effectively in real clinical scenarios. The theory, rooted in the ANS's responses to social and environmental cues, is a valuable tool for understanding and promoting overall patient well-being and safety. Research reveals that somatic psychology can provide healthcare professionals with evidence-based interventions focusing on the relationship between the mind and the body, thereby allowing them to treat certain mental health conditions, such as dissociative disorders (Reuille-Dupont 2020). Embracing the PVT in healthcare not only enhances risk assessment but also allows for a deeper comprehension of the physiological and psychological aspects of safety, ultimately leading to more holistic and patient-centered care strategies.

In our 2022 research paper, we contend that stress and trauma are major influences on a person's physiological responses and decision-making. Other researchers posit that stress and decision-making are intertwined in a complex relationship. For instance, Starcke and Brand (2012) argue that stress diverts cognitive resources away from the higher-order thinking process. Understanding the impacts of emotional influences such as stress and trauma allow healthcare professionals to determine appropriate recommendations for improving the patient's mental health and well-being.

The PVT also offers a range of practical techniques for regulating the ANS, which can be applied in mental health settings. Suitable examples include mindfulness-related and compassion-related meditations (Poli et al. 2021). These contemplative practices act as neural exercises that enhance the functioning of the VVC, a key component of the ANS responsible for promoting a state of calmness and social engagement. Recent research has demonstrated the effectiveness of these practices as health interventions for various medical conditions ranging from cardiovascular disease, posttraumatic stress disorder (PTSD), vascular disease, fibromyalgia, lower back pain, and hypertension to obsessive-compulsive disorder (OCD) (Poli et al. 2021). The connection between contemplative practices and vagal activation is significant because vagal activation is associated with a state of calmness and social engagement, which can have a profound impact on overall health and well-being. By integrating these techniques into mental healthcare, professionals can empower patients to self-regulate and manage stress, anxiety, and trauma-related symptoms effectively. By teaching individuals how to harness the power of their own nervous systems, clinicians can significantly improve their patients' mental health outcomes and overall quality of life.

Thrive, Not Just Survive

The PVT extends the concept of safety beyond the traditional boundaries of psychology and mental health. The theory recognizes that feelings of safety are not limited to emotional well-being but also encompass physical health, education, societal interactions, and other dimensions of life. In his article "Polyvagal Theory: A Science of Safety," Porges (2022, 11) states that "Feelings of safety play a fundamental role enabling humans not only to survive, but to thrive." For instance, he believes that incorporating PVT exercises into one's routines can help professionals cultivate essential skills such as resilience.

At its core, resilience involves a combination of behavioral, physiological, emotional, and social processes that allow the restoration of ANS function in support of the social engagement state (Porges 2022, 11). Based on the polyvagal perspective, resilience is not merely about bouncing back from adversity but also about re-establishing a physiological and emotional equilibrium that fosters positive social interactions with others and contributes to an individual's overall well-being. For that reason, the science of safety has significant implications in other branches of the healthcare industry, such as human resources and even facility layout and design.

Polyvagal-Informed Exercises to Explore and Regulate ANS Function

A person who spends most of their time in a ventral vagal state (the state of safety and socialization) tends to have a flexible range of emotions. They can generally operate in a sympathetic state as needed without setting off a cascade of excess of stress hormones such as cortisol. They can express themselves in a relaxed or charged situation. They can even argue and disagree without being in highly stressed states. They can be excited and/or engaged and then settle down as necessary. They can also be relaxed and engaged in conversation while sharing a meal with others, properly digesting their food and then resuming their tasks afterward.

The following polyvagal-informed exercises help you recalibrate your autonomic state to spend more time in this ideal state so that you can be productive and at ease and help others do the same. Although we cannot directly control our neuroception, we can build our interoceptive skills to understand where we are on the polyvagal ladder at any moment in time. This is the first step in building our capacity to influence our current state, thus growing our success in mitigating stress. As we become more resilient, both our job performance and our quality of life can improve.

Neuroception and Interoception Practice

Your brain's sensory cortex gathers information from the world around you and relays it through the thalamus to the amygdala. The amygdala can act as an alarm center in the brain when there is a perceived or real threat to safety, but it is also important in registering salient or important emotional information. The amygdala will signal the hypothalamic-pituitary-adrenal (HPA) axis to release cortisol, adrenaline, and other hormones to gear your SNS toward protective action. When a threat is over, the amygdala conversely signals the brain that it can stand down. With these exercises, you provide your sensory cortex with information that you choose in order to short circuit the initial threat response where no real threat exists to return more quickly to a state of calm.

You would likely agree that most of us are generally safe at work. And while some level of sympathetic activation is required to perform our tasks, it should not be so intense as to engage our survival physiology. Neuroception and interoception practices can help you decrease unneeded high sympathetic arousal or, when necessary, help you shift out of dorsal vagal shutdown.

Using your perception of sight, sound, touch, smell, and taste to identify safety, your sense of neuroception provides your ANS with a cue of "safeness," which then provides internal cues of safety, leading to feelings of confidence and well-being – even during difficult and/or challenging experiences.

The following exercises access polyvagal structures (the ventral vagal, sympathetic, and dorsal vagal pathways) directly and engage processes that are usually unconscious. Not having these tools is one reason why many intelligent people are overstressed and are unable to think their way out of their symptoms and problems. It doesn't have to be this way.

> **Caution:** *These skills are meant to be practiced by recalling a stressful memory in an effort to change how your nervous system will respond in future stressful situations. If something dangerous or threatening IS occurring in your environment, your body SHOULD respond through the activation of the SNS. You can process that experience later using polyvagal-informed approaches.*

Exercise A: Directly Engage Neuroception for Cues of Safety

These exercises are best performed when you are under no perceived threat or danger, allowing you time to learn the skills. As you progress in your practice, you can then begin to use them during moments of stress to help increase your resilience. You can use one or more of your senses to orient yourself to your environment, thereby directly engaging neuroception and providing your ANS with external cues of safety to help restore a sense of productive calm. "Safety" may be something you like, something neutral, something stable, or something simply nonthreatening.

You can do these sensory exercises without much movement, so they can be performed right in the moment. Here are some ideas for engaging each of your senses:

- **Visual/Sight:** What do you see? Notice colors, textures, objects, and qualities. Perhaps your eyes are drawn to a window, a plant, a coffee cup, a carpet pattern, or the wood of the desk. In a hospital setting, perhaps you are drawn to the symmetry of a medical device, a kind way someone is interacting with a patient, or the color of the scrubs you chose. Are there things in the space you are drawn to or interested in? Allow your eyes to settle there for a few moments. **Tip:** If there's normally little visual stimuli in your environment, you can wear something appealing (a certain color, for instance) that you can focus on visually as needed to reorient yourself.
- **Auditory/Hearing:** What do you hear? Listen for the sound of familiar voices, perhaps of people with whom you have a good working relationship. This is less about what they say and more about the cadence and tone of their voice in your ear. Listen, too, for simple sounds like the rhythm of your footsteps or the click of a keyboard. Maybe there is music playing somewhere you can tune into. If you are outside or a window is open, can you hear the wind or birds, or even traffic rushing by? If it is quiet, perhaps you can tune into the steady hum of a machine. Simply listen for a few moments.
- **Tactile/Feeling:** What can you feel? Run your hand across the fabric of your clothing or take some time to notice how it feels against your skin. Touch a surface, such as the wood or metal of a chair; it might feel solid under your hand or cool. You can place your hand on your other hand or on your forehead, noticing the texture and temperature of your skin. Experience the tactile sensations for a few moments.
- **Gustatory/Taste:** What do you taste? Perhaps you recently ate something, and the flavor is lingering or perhaps you just popped a mint or brushed your teeth. If you have a water bottle or other drink with you, take a sip and notice the taste. Perhaps run your tongue along your lips, noticing the subtle taste. **Tip:** Some people find that eating or drinking can be stabilizing. Tea, water, or other healthy drinks and snacks are good choices. If this is you, make sure that you are not "stress eating" to force your system into a calmer state. Rather, eat or drink something small, while being mindful of the taste and attentive to flavor.
- **Olfactory/Smell:** What do you smell? Perhaps you've chosen a pleasant-smelling shampoo or deodorant that day. Spend a few moments noticing its appealing scent. If you are a scent-oriented person, perhaps you can sniff from a favorite, calming essential oil bottle for a moment of aromatherapy (there is more on aromatherapy in Chapter 6). **Note:** When a scent is inhaled, it is not relayed through the thalamus but goes directly to the amygdala (where emotional memory is registered). This can be particularly helpful for someone who is dissociated (i.e., disconnected from oneself). Scent can be used to reconnect with the body or present moment. Aromatherapy is a simple way to bring a higher level of presence and nervous system regulation.

Exercise B: Engage Interoception for Cues of Safety

Internal neuroception of danger is usually an internal sensation like pain, emptiness, constriction, a "charge" or burst of energy, and discomfort. This is brought to conscious awareness by the process of interoception. Your mind will lock into these states to try to figure out how to resolve them, which is a useful process when there is a real problem but a nuisance when there is no real threat or stressor. When we improve our interoceptive skill and begin to use regulation exercises for our nervous system, we can begin to reduce how often our neuroception triggers a "false alarm." This leads to improved resilience and stress levels. There are several techniques to work with an internal sense of danger. Let's take a look at two step-by-step options to begin. We'll share a few others later in the book.

Advanced training: Consider working with a NeuroConsulting Group training team for live educational sessions. For more information, see the concluding chapter.

Option 1

1. Tune into your body for signals of internal stress. This could be a sensation of tightness, heat or cold, a racing heart, or rapid breathing, for example.
2. Become aware of the sensations you feel in this moment and describe them to yourself.
3. Connect to external cues of safety (see Exercise B) and orient to them for as long as you feel you need to (for most, this takes up to 30 seconds).
4. Tune back into your body to see if those external cues of safety changed your interoceptive sense of safety. If you don't notice a change, repeat the steps. If this still doesn't work, revisit this practice when you're in a calmer environment.
5. Continue connecting to external cues of safety as you go about your tasks.

Here is an example:

> Dr. Jennings feels tight in her chest. She becomes aware that the tightness is located in her upper chest and shoulders. It feels like a taut rubber band. She takes a moment to look out the window. She sees a tree swaying in the wind and silvery-green leaves falling to the ground. As she watches, she checks back into the feeling in her chest. It feels less tight. Dr. Jennings takes a moment to enjoy feeling looser.
>
> Dr. Jennings knows there will be some tension today because she has a lot to do. She needs some sympathetic energy to get through the day. But she is more at ease now and feels less overwhelmed. Dr. Jennings goes to her next task. As she is walking, she listens to the sound of her footsteps and feels her feet. When she sees the patient, the patient's mother is gently holding her hand. Dr. Jennings takes in this sight and feels touched. The interoception of "touched" in this moment manifests as a little more softening of the tension in her chest, and her shoulders soften slightly, too.
>
> When Dr. Jennings hears about the patient's traumatic injury, she feels her chest tightening again. But when the sharing is complete, Dr. Jennings sits on the stool to enter her notes. Next to the computer is a pen holder from her alma mater. She looks at it briefly, remembering her experience there and how her education will be instrumental in helping this patient. Some of the tension releases.

Option 2

1. Tune into your body for signals of internal stress. This could be a sensation of tightness, heat or cold, a racing heart or rapid breathing, for example.
2. Become aware of the sensations you feel in this moment and describe them to yourself.
3. Move your attention to a place in your body that is *not* feeling the "negative" sensation.
4. Spend some time focusing on the area that does not feel the "negative" sensation. Do not pay attention to the negative sensation while still tending to your awareness of being

in your body. Keep your attention on the area(s) that feel pleasant or neutral. In essence, you are cultivating an awareness that "not everything is bad" in your body.
5. Holding the more positive experience in your awareness, return your attention to the location of the sensation of stress you identified. Notice if there is any change. It's OK if there is no change yet. If this occurs, you can simply return to focusing on the sensation that is pleasant or neutral, and then recheck your area where you feel stress.
6. Alternatively, hold both the positive interoceptive and negative interoceptive experiences in your awareness at the same time. You might need to do this for several seconds to a minute or two. It often won't change immediately, as this part of the nervous system is slow to respond.

Here's an example:

> Dr. Jennings has tension in her shoulders and a feeling of worry. She feels the tension across her upper shoulders but notices it does not spread to her mid-back. The feeling of worry is a fluttery feeling in her chest and a heavy feeling in her stomach.
>
> As she walks between her office and the cafeteria, she moves her attention to her legs, which feel strong and steady. She spends a few minutes taking in the quality of this pleasant sensation. As she turns the corner, she brings her attention back to her stomach and shoulders. The fluttery feelings have lessened and she feels lighter. She focuses not just on the absence of tightness or heaviness but on the increase in softness and ease. Alternatively, she could have noticed her legs, stomach, and shoulders all at the same time, allowing plenty of time for sensory changes.
>
> By the time Dr. Jennings walks into the cafeteria, she realizes how hungry she is. She is also more aware of the people around her and decides to sit with a colleague instead of eating alone as she had planned.

Social-Engagement Awareness Practice

Direct positive social-engagement experiences can engage polyvagal structures to increase the capacity of the ventral vagal state. Just as you would exercise a muscle at the gym, practicing social engagement skills directly increases your ability to connect with others. As a quick reminder, the PVT teaches us that we are hardwired to connect and that this is a biological mandate for our survival. The following two exercises, which are essentially awareness exercises, can easily be incorporated into any safe environment and practiced throughout the day.

Exercise C: Awareness of Interoception During Social Interactions

When you are engaged in a pleasant social interaction, bring your attention to your sense of interoception. You do not have to stop what you're doing. Throughout your day, simply take notice of the following:

- What sensations do you experience in your body when you laugh with your colleagues or a patient?
- What happens in your body when you listen to someone speaking about an interesting topic?
- What qualities in your body do you notice when you hear kind words or expressions of gratitude?

Exercise D: Awareness of Nonverbal Cues of Safety

There are many nonverbal cues of safety in an environment, such as a wave, smile, or simple contact such as a pat on the back. Even someone moving a chair out of your way is an opportunity to recognize well-intentioned gestures. The majority of these moments often go unseen or unrecognized on a conscious level. However, if you make an effort to become more aware of these cues of safety on a conscious level, you can experience the positive effects on your emotions and physiology.

Throughout your day, take note of the following:
- Pleasant facial expressions such as a smile, nod of approval, or an interested gaze.
- Friendly gestures such as a wave or a firm handshake.
- Kind acts, such as someone holding the door open for you or even serving you a meal.

As you experience these nonverbal cues of safely, become aware of your sense of interoception. How do these acts affect your physiology? Increasing awareness of physiological states with cues of safety increases your ventral vagal capacity. The more you practice being in a ventral vagal state, the more access you have to emotional and physical well-being. In this state, you can be more productive, be a better problem-solver and team player, and give greater assistance to others.

Here is an example:

> Amanda Vincent, RN, one of the staff nurses who has undergone the PVT training with Dr. Jennings, arrived at the office feeling tired. She had a hectic morning, and her car just broke down in the parking lot. At least she'd made it to work. When she enters the office, she notices her colleague's warm smile. "Good morning, Amanda," her colleague, Lisa, says from behind the desk.
>
> Amanda registers the smile and notices she feels some relief. She hadn't been aware of pain in her shoulders until it lets go a little.
>
> "How are you doing today?" Lisa asks while taking notes.
>
> "My car just died, in the lot," says Amanda. "And I was on the phone with my bank half the morning clearing up a strange withdrawal. I'm pretty stressed." As she is speaking, Amanda notices that she feels a little softer and some of the agitation she felt is settling down in her chest. But she's still worried about her car and how the rest of the day will go with that problem weighing on her mind.
>
> "I can help you with that," Lisa says, looking up from her work, making eye contact with Amanda. "My cousin runs a towing service nearby and could help you out."
>
> Amanda feels more tension release from her shoulders. She notices she is able to take a deeper breath. She thought she might have to wait until the end of the day to call a tow truck. It was going to be a late night. "I'll take you up on that, thank you," she says and swipes her badge to head into work.
>
> Many patients are already in the waiting room. Amanda is walking toward a desk and notices her body. She feels slightly hopeful that the day will go more smoothly. Her heart rate has decreased, and she's feeling more settled. There's still some stress, but she feels touched by her colleague's support and relieved that some action will be taken.

Exercise E: Engage Your Middle Ear

This exercise engages the middle ear when you listen to the sounds of voices around you. Muscles in the middle ear modulate the frequencies our brains focus on, with an emphasis on lower frequency sounds when neuroception perceives a possible threat. Experts in the field have developed sound-based therapies in an effort to help infuse the brain with cues of safety, thus shifting the nervous system from dorsal vagal or sympathetic states to a more connected ventral vagal state. By paying attention to sounds, you may notice both how sounds affect you as well as how your internal interoceptive state can change your hearing (by triggering the focus on possible danger).

See if you can tune in not to the words that someone is speaking, but to the musicality or the cadence in a person's voice. Listen to the tone of the person's voice as a vibration. Particularly tune into voices of people that you like and connect with well. For example, if you show your badge at reception and your colleague greets you, the sound of that person's voice might increase your neuroception of safety. If it does, then also notice the corresponding sensations in your body that tell you that you feel safe or OK.

Stimulating Your VVC

As mentioned, the VVC is a set of pathways that are activated when we feel safe, allowing us to connect socially to others. Some days we're not feeling particularly social, which is okay unless we are in a setting where we must interact with others, such as when we are at work. In cases like that, you can use polyvagal-informed techniques such as the sympathetic exercises (see section on "SNS Strategies") or dorsal vagal exercises (see section on "Dorsal Vagal Strategies") to shift to a ventral vagal state. However, another quick way to help you reset your circuitry to the ventral vagal state is by stimulating your VVC.

From a neuroanatomical standpoint, when you wake up this pathway through use, you stimulate the VVC. Flip back to Figure 1.1 diagraming the cranial nerves as part of the VVC; many of these nerves are involved in facial and eye movements.

- **Head, neck, and eyes:** Look around the room, fully engaging your head, neck, and eyes, without consciously directing them. Allow them to move at will. Permit soft movements to engage the back of your skull, as well, especially if you're feeling tight back there. Try to allow the movement to come from the inside rather than moving them the way you think you should. If this instruction seems foreign to you, which it might, any kind of movement will be helpful. As you move, notice if you start to feel more awareness of your environment, greater presence of your body, or more alert.
- **Face:** Lightly massage your face. Alternatively, scrunch your face, stretch, and release; consider face yoga exercises. Try to feel your face from the outside and/or inside. Children naturally express emotions on their faces. As adults, we tend to keep our primal emotions under a "socially acceptable" mask. However, we should not allow the tone of our facial muscles to become dormant, rigid, or slack. Flexing your facial muscles, as instructed, engages structures involved in social engagement. When you are done with the facial movements, allow your face to express an emotion you are experiencing. Notice if this helps you feel more alert, present, settled, or active. **Tip:** When appropriate and you are with trusted others, practice allowing more emotional expression to come to your face so that they can read and respond to your emotional state appropriately.

SNS Strategies

The SNS is responsible for any state of excitation, including states of negative stress, positive stress, and positive excitement. The following exercises can be used to decrease negative stress (a common complaint in the workplace), modulate positive stress, and increase or more fully enjoy states of positive excitement.

Exercise F: Decreasing Negative Stress

1. Bring any stress you are feeling to your interceptive awareness, even if it is subtle right now. (When you can identify lower levels of stress, you are in a better position to thwart further dysregulation and distress.)
2. Become aware of the area in your body where you feel the stress. Is it in your forehead or face, chest, arms, belly, legs, or elsewhere?
3. If you feel tension in your body, go to the edge of that tension pattern by literally seeing if you can detect where the tension goes away in your body, as if the area of tension has a shape to it, and notice if anything changes on its own. Alternatively, place your hand over the area of tension and wait for a few minutes to see if it decreases.
4. Wait for your breath to come naturally; don't consciously breathe into the area. Move your attention to a nearby area of your body that feels better or less intense. By placing your hand over the top of the area of tension, you can see if anything changes on its own.

Note: It is a frequent observation that touch can settle the nervous system, just as a mother holds a baby to soothe it. Likewise, "self-holding" stimulates a deep reorganization from the SNS to provide relief.

Exercise G: Modulate Positive Stress Exercises

Sometimes, we can be highly productive, engaged, and focused, but even then we might need to let off energy to ensure that this positive stress doesn't lead to a heightened sympathetic activation. You can think of this exercise as an adrenaline dump. Ignoring this cycle perpetuates ongoing cycles of sympathetic activation in the nervous system. To release the energy naturally, follow these steps:

1. When you feel positive stress, take some time to notice that you are "amped up" and how that manifests for you physiologically (e.g., heat, vibration, tingling, etc.). Is there a different quality of sensation with positive stress compared to negative stress?
2. Acknowledge that this feeling is in relationship to things you want to do or is connected to positive motivation in your life and work.
3. Notice the capacity of your physical body to hold this charge. Feel the width of your hips, your back, your shoulder blades, and your ribcage providing a sense of support or containment for the charge.
4. Observe how the adrenaline moves through your body. For example, perhaps you notice the way heat shifts from your core to your periphery or how the vibration or tingling travels. Staying with the feeling of the movement of the adrenaline shifting through your body will help you fully release it. As you observe, notice how the feeling naturally decreases with awareness.

Tip: When you feel a positive stress charge that's building too swiftly, place your focus downward – for instance, notice the sensations of your feet on the floor or your backside on a chair. Feel the movement downward from your brain through your body. This can decrease some of the SNS charge while keeping your body energized and engaged.

Exercise H: Enjoy States of Positive Excitement

The SNS is not only associated with fight-or-flight responses. Mobilization includes pleasant experiences of play (e.g., enjoying a good game of tennis). When combined with an activated VVC, the SNS helps us connect with others in both intimate and group settings. While a pure ventral vagal state may be more akin to relaxed socialization, the addition of sympathetic energy introduces excitement and movement. In our journey of understanding our own nervous systems, it's helpful to be able to identify positive sympathetic states.

1. Remember a time when you were having a lot of fun with others, perhaps playing a game, laughing in an energetic meeting, or engaging in a fun physical activity.
2. As you recall this time, begin to notice how your body is responding in the current moment, building your interoception skills.
3. When you recall how you felt good, notice the sensations in your body now. What happens in your face, throat, chest, belly, arms, and legs? Do you feel heavier or lighter? Do you feel like moving? Do you feel any energy, tingling, or warmth?
4. Let the feeling of the positive states show in your facial expression; see if you can allow your face to express what you're feeling inside. When you smile, feel the expansion in your chest that occurs along with it. If laughter arises, enjoy how it feels.
5. As you feel excited and good, notice if you can feel a pleasant charge inside your body – like electricity, flow, warmth, or light. Enjoy the feelings and sensations.

Dorsal Vagal Strategies

The prior exercises generally focused on shifting to the ventral vagal state from a state of sympathetic activation. Without some modulation, sympathetic activation has the potential to shift down to the dorsal vagal state (the bottom rung of the polyvagal ladder), rather than upward (to the top rung of the ladder). Because this is an experience of extreme collapse, exhaustion, depression, and/or lack of motivation, the dorsal vagal state is one of the hardest places to shift from; there's a lot weighing us down. Here are a few ways to lighten the load and climb up and out of this state of immobilization:

1. **Sigh or make a sound that expresses how you are feeling.** Sigh all the way to the end of your out breath and allow a deeper, fuller breath to come in after. Alternatively, hum for 30 seconds, noticing the vibration in your mouth, throat, and body. Once you have done this, bring your awareness to your sense of interoception. Notice if you're feeling any better or more engaged. Do you sense more vibration or aliveness? A little more energized? A little more relaxed? A little bit more motivated or directed toward your next task? As with prior exercises, if you don't notice a shift the first time, try it again once or twice. If that doesn't create a shift, don't despair. Simply move on to a different exercise.
2. **Move to counteract immobility.** Stand up and scrunch your toes. Rotate your ankles one at a time. Then progress upward to your knees, hips, spine, shoulders, elbows, wrists, and fingers, gently rotating each joint. If you must remain seated, you can shift your state more subtly by rotating your ankles under your desk. Save vigorous movement for after you have unthawed from the dorsal vagal state, allowing for gradual change. Following lockdown or shut-off mode, you may have to deal a task you had been too collapsed to handle. When you have more energy, try one of the SNS or ventral vagal exercises given earlier in this chapter.

3. **Orient to specific objects.** The "head, neck, and eyes" exercise (Exercise F) is a good strategy for shifting from dorsal vagal states, but it may be more helpful to orient to specific objects around you. In visual orienting, do you see anything you can sense into (i.e., as you observe an object, notice any change in your bodily sensations – ideally, sensations that produce settling or calming). With tactile orienting, notice, for example, if your clothing is smooth or rough. Pairing your touch receptors with the present moment can disrupt dorsal vagal physiology because your ANS is now attending to new inputs that are neutral or pleasant.
4. **Try tapping.** Tapping areas of your body with your fingers is a technique that is used in several types of therapy, including Emotional Freedom Technique (EFT). Tapping is one way to bring back a sense of your body having distinct boundaries and being self-contained. It also increases circulation to the area you are tapping. It usually increases a neutral to pleasant sense of connection to your body. You do not need to tap any particular place or in a particular pattern, only in a way that you find might helpful to you.

ANS Regulation Strategies to Effect Internal Change

The exercises provided so far are an excellent starting place for enhancing your self-awareness, allowing you to work more effectively, both with yourself and with others. The following exercises help reduce cumulative stress and increase your ventral vagal capacity.

Exercise I: The Photograph

The name of this exercise harkens back to the process of developing photographs. Unlike digital photography, in analog photography it takes time for a photograph to develop – that is, for an image to emerge. Paying attention to your polyvagal state and watching how it develops, or changes, is called "somatic reprisal." With this conscious attention, the state will generally develop toward regulation – or up the ladder.

1. Place your conscious attention on your internal state. Notice any sensations that arise in your conscious awareness. For example, look at areas where you may feel light or heavy, warm or cool, tingly or numb, tense or relaxed.
2. As if waiting in a darkroom, watch your identified sensation as it develops into something clearer. The more you pay attention, the more specific sensations will emerge. The sensation may also shift to a different area in the body or change in quality.
3. Notice if your internal sensory photograph develops toward regulation – that is, whether you notice feeling calmer or more connected to yourself and/or others. If this does not occur, don't despair. You can repeat the exercise once or twice, or simply move back to the previous exercises. This process can take time and produce varied results, so do not worry if your results are different.

Exercise J: ANS Regulation Protocols

The ANS Regulation Protocols help you regulate your ANS to increase your ventral vagal capacity. There's an example following the protocols to show how you can use this protocol for yourself. Once you become familiar with them yourself, you can teach these protocols to others, such as patients, colleagues, and employees.

Protocol 1: The Shift

This is a reprisal or a shift of state, hopefully more toward regulation or ventral vagal tone. When we find ourselves in a dorsal vagal or sympathetic state, but with no danger present, we typically want the ability to guide our nervous system back to a more ventral vagal state. This will reduce our stress overall and improve our sense of well-being.

1. **Notice and name:** Identify where you are on the polyvagal ladder. Check in to see if there is a location of the PVT state in your body (is it in your shoulders or chest, for example?) Is there one or more sensations in that area of your body? For example, you may notice tension in your neck, which suggests you are in a SNS state of tension or bracing. Or you may notice a dull feeling in the pit of your stomach, which hints at a dorsal vagal state of collapse.
2. **Watch and wait:** As you notice the sensation you identified, just wait and observe it. Frequently, the sensation will begin to change and shift on its own, without you needing to "do" anything. For example, if you noticed tension in your neck, simply observe the tension and see if something changes. This step typically takes a minute or two, so don't rush and take your time. If nothing happens, you can check back and notice another sensation in your body and observe that instead, or you may simply prefer to stop the exercise and try something different.
3. **Change:** Keep your attention directed toward any change you may notice. Identify what changes. Even small shifts are important; you can then track whether the sensation moves to another area of your body or stays in the same place but changes in quality. This is similar to mindful observation. For example, if you have tension in your neck, observing it may lead to the tension reducing, disappearing, or even moving to a different area of your body. Again, if this does not happen, don't worry. You can repeat these steps or try a different exercise.

Protocol 2: The Switch

1. **Notice and name:** Identify where you are on the polyvagal ladder. Check in to see if there is a location of the PVT state in your body (is it in your shoulders or chest, for example?) Is there one or more sensation(s) in that area of your body? For example, you may notice tension in your neck, which suggests you are in a SNS state of tension or bracing. Or you may notice a dull feeling in the pit of your stomach, which hints at a dorsal vagal state of collapse.
2. **Watch and wait:** As with the previous exercise, take a minute or two to mindfully observe the sensation you identified. Do not try to change or shift the sensation (e.g., trying to relax a tense muscle).
3. **Change:** Just as before, look out for any shift or change in the sensation that may arise. Even small shifts are important. Name the change to yourself. If you were feeling heavy in one part of your body, for example, you may notice it feels a bit lighter just with being observed.
4. **Switch attention:** Switch attention to a regulation tool, such as orienting visually to your surroundings, humming, or noticing your feet on the ground, and notice how that helps. If it doesn't help, simply go back to observing the sensation and try again to see if it shifts or changes. If that doesn't seem to help after one or two more tries, you can try a different exercise.

5. **Return to change:** After you use the regulation tool of your choice, go back to observing the sensation in your body and track for any changes in quality, intensity, or location. In the example of a tense neck, switching attention could lead to relaxation in the neck, and as you return to change, you can then see if the relaxation moves anywhere else in the body or even whether any tension returns somewhere. Again, don't worry if this doesn't happen every time you try this.

Here is an example:

> Amanda Vincent, RN, is feeling tired. She's plodding along the hall with heavy eyelids, getting sleepier with each step. She wonders how she'll be able to get through the meeting she'll be heading into in a few minutes. Then she remembers the Shift Protocol.
>
> As she continues on her way, she silently asks herself, "What is my polyvagal state?" She identifies that she in in the dorsal vagal state, the bottom rung of the ladder. "Where and how do I feel that?" She checks in with herself and thinks, "My chest feels heavy, and my feet feel like clay ... I'll watch and wait."
>
> Amanda stays with the feeling and realizes the heaviness spreads <u>and that she feels more of it in her belly</u>. As she does this, she feels a little less pressure in her chest. This causes her to roll her shoulders a bit and automatically breathe more deeply. Noticing that she feels a little more awake, she decides to use the Switch Protocol, too, and starts looking around as she walks. The hall is lit with glaring florescent lights, but the marble pattern on the floor reminds her of a visually pleasing statue she saw at a museum on Saturday. She looks at the marble pattern and recalls the statue.
>
> After a few moments, she checks back into her chest and feet, and they feel a little more energized. As she approaches the conference room door, she notes that she still feels tired but is more ready to fully participate in the meeting.

Key Takeaways

- The PVT originated from the pioneering work of Dr. Stephen Porges and holds profound relevance in understanding mental health. Porges built upon the foundations laid by earlier well-known scholars such as Charles Darwin, John Hughlings Jackson, and Paul MacLean, who explored the mind–body connection and the role of the vagus nerve in physiological responses. Porges's key contribution was recognizing the evolutionary significance of the ANS in regulating social behavior and responses to stress. Understanding this theory helps healthcare professionals effectively address issues such as anxiety, stress, and social engagement with polyvagal-informed exercises.
- The PVT conceptualizes the ANS as a dynamic system with three distinct states responsible for regulating various physiological and behavioral responses based on one's perceptions of safety or threat. Foremost, the VVC is a branch of the parasympathetic nerve that aims to prevent overactivity and support social interactions. The VVC usually strengthens the socialization state. In comparison, the SNS is a separate branch of the ANS primarily responsible for preparing the body to respond to threats. The SNS tends to support mobilization through the flight-or-fight response. The DVC is another branch of the PNS that tends to slow down the heart rate and conserve metabolic resources during extreme stress or threat. This pathway is usually associated with immobilization.
- Understanding these core components is essential for applying the PVT in clinical practice to gain insight into various mental health issues. When people are in a high

sympathetic state of mobilization or dorsal vagal shutdown, productivity and satisfaction often plummet. Another way to look at this is that there is survival physiology, a baseline that is taking away people's attention from being creative and connected in the workplace. It also keeps some from feeling their best self. When we feel capable and in control (i.e., when we are in the ventral vagal state), we tend to engage within our own inner thoughts, and with others', collaboratively and curiously.

- The polyvagal ladder provides a reliable framework for visualizing the three states of the ANS. When one is feeling safe and connected with others, they are on the top rung of the ladder. In this state, the person is likely to engage in positive social interaction. However, when faced with a triggering situation, they shift down to the middle of the ladder, which is marked by specific physiological responses that trigger the fight-or-flight response. If the situation becomes too overwhelming, they drop down to the bottom rung of the ladder: immobilization.
- The PVT aligns with the advancements in modern health research that have allowed for a deeper understanding of the neural mechanisms underlying the ANS and its impact on mental health. In addition, the theory offers a practical framework for strengthening somatic (body-centered) psychology by bridging the gap between the mind and body. The theory has also transformed the understanding of how stress and trauma affect physiological processes and decision-making. Another potential contribution lies in the use of polyvagal-informed techniques that strengthen social engagement among individuals.
- Developing your interoception, or the awareness of your own autonomic state, and learning how to influence your physiology to be able to shift to a more regulated state as needed is an essential first step in effecting positive change in the healthcare industry.

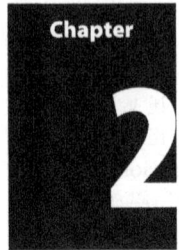

Chapter 2: Developing ANS-Focused Clinical Interventions

Now that we've explored some of the core concepts of the PVT, we can turn our attention to how to implement our understanding in the services provided to our customers, whether we identify them as patients, clients, or whatever is the accepted norm for your organization and community. This can include both general medical and behavioral health specialty organizations. In this chapter, we present a structured guide on the integration of the PVT into clinical practice for healthcare practitioners. We start by highlighting the obstacles facing the integration of somatic (body-focused) psychology into clinical practice. Then we review various polyvagal-informed interventions that can improve patient health and well-being. The chapter also narrows down the clinical measures that can be used to assess the outcomes of polyvagal-informed interventions.

Objectives

- To identify the challenges and opportunities facing the integration of the PVT in psychology by healthcare professionals.
- To explain various clinical interventions that rely on polyvagal-informed techniques to improve patient health and well-being.
- To compare different clinical measures for evaluating the outcomes of polyvagal-informed interventions.

Integrating the PVT in Healthcare

Fundamentally, the challenges and opportunities affecting the integration of the PVT in healthcare stem from the wide divide between cognitive psychology and somatic psychology. Cognitive (mind-oriented) psychology and somatic (or body-oriented) psychology represent two distinct fields of psychology, with cognitive psychology still being the more popular of the two. Since the PVT aligns more closely with the principles of somatic psychology, many cognitive psychologists may struggle to incorporate polyvagal-informed interventions in their practice.

Somatic psychology emerged as a significant departure from the traditional cognitive psychology paradigm (Barratt 2010). That said, some researchers contend that somatic psychology is merely an extension of cognitive psychology, as it seeks to broaden its scope to incorporate a novel subject area (Barratt 2010, 5). Nevertheless, cognitive psychology, which predominantly focuses on dissecting internal cognitive structures and functions to decipher human behaviors, prioritizes an individual's internal factors as the key to achieving "scientific progress" (Barratt 2010, 13). This progress is often measured by the discipline's ability to manipulate, predict, and control human behavior from a cognitive perspective, relegating the body to an inferior role that passively responds to internal factors and external environmental variables in the process of regulating behaviors.

With the emergence of somatic psychology and body–mind therapy, the field of psychology embarked on a potentially revolutionary journey toward a better understanding of the human condition. Simply stated, in contrast to cognitive psychology, somatic psychology underlines the significance of the body and its intricate connection with psychological well-being. This departure from cognitive psychology is rooted in the acknowledgment of the complex interplay between the body and the mind. Instead of solely focusing on internal cognitive processes and structures, somatic psychology recognizes the body as a vital component in understanding human behavior and mental health.

With regard to the PVT, people who experience traumatic situations are often pushed beyond their physical and mental capacities. As a result, these events can trigger stress, anxiety, and other mental health conditions. Although cognitive-behavioral interventions are often used to support patients with mental health issues, the reality is that many individuals who experience traumatic situations tend to show impaired somatic functioning. This can include decreased coordination, gastrointestinal problems, migraine headaches, elevated heart rate and palpitations, and increased incidence of skin disorders linked to inflammatory conditions. In fact, research reveals that cognitive psychology is inadequate for explaining and addressing the neurophysiological impacts of stress and trauma (Vanderpal and Brazie 2022).

Somatic psychology has emerged as a popular strategy for strengthening the link between the body and the mind. This function is controlled by the subcortical brain systems, and they usually aim to change how the body responds to trauma and other adverse mental experiences. For instance, *somatic experiencing* (SE) is a promising intervention for mitigating mental health symptoms that stem from traumatic experiences. According to SE theory, posttraumatic stress symptoms often arise from the body's failure to complete its natural response to stress during the traumatic event (Kuhfuß et al. 2021). Therefore, somatic psychology interventions are integral for addressing such issues and helping individuals strengthen their resilience toward surrounding threats, and for reducing the tendency to perceive threats when none exist.

To effectively integrate the PVT into healthcare, a paradigm shift needs to occur within the field, recognizing the significance of somatic psychology and the body–mind connection. This shift involves acknowledging that mental health and well-being cannot be fully understood or addressed without considering the somatic aspects of human experience. By bridging the gap between cognitive and somatic perspectives, healthcare professionals can develop more holistic and comprehensive approaches for improving patient outcomes and promoting overall well-being.

The Challenge of Employing the PVT in Clinical Practice

One of the central challenges faced by Dr. Jennings's team involved the integration of the PVT into their clinical practice. Since the theory focuses primarily on somatic psychology rather than cognitive psychology, many staff members were unsure how to use the concepts with their patients. This change requires Dr. Jennings and her team to re-evaluate existing therapeutic practices and adapt to a more holistic understanding of mental health that focuses more on the connection between the body and the mind.

Dr. Jennings took the initiative to educate her team about the PVT, concentrating on its relevance to mental health and effective strategies for incorporating polyvagal-informed interventions to enhance patients' health and well-being. Using Fred Johnson's case as a model, Dr. Jennings illustrated the practical application of the PVT in their clinical practice. This transformative shift necessitates a reassessment of existing therapeutic approaches, urging Dr. Jennings and her team to embrace a more comprehensive understanding of mental health that emphasizes the intricate connection between the body and the mind. By providing her team with insight into these clinical interventions and assessment measures, Dr. Jennings intends to empower them to deliver comprehensive and effective care to patients grappling with issues related to fear, stress, and anxiety.

As a result, Dr. Jennings opted to implement various evidence-based interventions aligned with the PVT. These interventions include self-regulation, interoception, SE, and aromatherapy. In addition, it was essential to consider whether group interventions could improve the patients' sense of safety. Another important topic involved strategies for using cues of safety to create an environment that exudes safety to patients as well as workers. Furthermore, Dr. Jennings and her team needed to understand how to use different clinical measures to evaluate the outcomes of these interventions. Using Fred Johnson as the first subject, Dr. Jennings compared various clinical measures: objective measures, subjective reports, behavioral observations, and standardized psychological assessments (see Chapter 5). By equipping her team with an understanding of these clinical interventions and assessment measures, Dr. Jennings aims to empower them to provide more holistic and effective care to patients grappling with fear, stress, and anxiety-related issues.

Steps for Implementing Polyvagal-Informed Interventions in the Healthcare Setting

Despite various limitations hindering the adoption of the PVT in modern healthcare, the theory offers the healthcare sector a significant opportunity to improve upon patient care and worker satisfaction. In essence, this approach is beneficial in several different ways: healthcare workers become more resilient and experience less stress and burnout, thus increasing productivity; leaders and managers become more effective and supportive; patients and their identified support persons will feel safer and more respected and listened to; and underlying mental health conditions can improve due to reduced anxiety, fear, and/or anger, which typically are associated with increased sympathetic or dorsal vagal states. The design and implementation of polyvagal-informed interventions encompass an interconnected series of approaches, broken down into seven key steps.

Step 1: Education

The first step is to educate healthcare workers and, ultimately, patients on the basic principles of the PVT. This empowers employees and patients by providing them with valuable insight on the three autonomic states and the factors that compel a person to shift between them. This insight gives them the foundation for the application of polyvagal-informed strategies.

Teaching these concepts is a remarkable opportunity to cause a shift in society's cognitive perspectives by encouraging people to think critically beyond the observable world (Hays 2019), essentially encouraging them to redefine their neural perceptions to better comprehend how information stored within the intricacies of the observable world unfolds. Being educated on the core components of the PVT provides a more solid understanding of the relationship between the body and the mind – that is, how our physiology affects our psychology.

What's more, the PVT introduces a fresh perspective for understanding impaired social behavior, which can manifest in various ways, from extreme to subtle. It underscores that an individual's physiological state significantly limits the range of their social interactions. Hence, there's a possibility that by inducing states of calmness and actively practicing the neural regulation of brainstem structures, it is possible to positively enhance social behavior and the benefits thereof, including increased happiness; less stress, irritability, and anxiety; and reduced stress on the body. It is well-known that people who are more socially connected tend to live longer and experience a better quality of life.

This particular viewpoint, which centers on behaviors rooted in biology, could be seen as a novel approach for modifying behavior – a fourth paradigm, so to speak. The three traditionally recognized paradigms are categorized according to behavioral (influenced by learning theory), biochemical (relying on pharmacological methods), and psychotherapeutic (encompassing psychoanalysis and cognitive therapies) intervention strategies (Porges 2003). Through this new, fourth lens, there are diverse opportunities to enhance social engagement and overall well-being with polyvagal-informed interventions.

Step 2: Map the ANS

Mapping the ANS and its respective states holds immense potential for strengthening a person's self-awareness and mental and emotional well-being. Self-awareness is essential to recognize when one is in a state of socialization/safety (ventral vagal), when one is experiencing stress or mobilization (sympathetic), or when one is in a state of shutdown (dorsal vagal). This knowledge empowers the person to make informed choices about how to regulate their responses to stressors. Mapping can also help identify the "triggers" that push them into a state of distress, as well as moments of resilience, or "glimmers," that promote safety and social engagement.

Autonomic mapping includes three established worksheets: the Personal Profile Map (Figure 2.1; shared earlier in Chapter 1), the Triggers and Glimmers Map (Figure 2.2), and the Regulating Resources Map (Figure 2.3), each of which we explore next. While the maps can be used by an individual, they are often used in group settings where communication is encouraged to deepen the practice and increase awareness.

> **Group Work**
>
> In the group setting, the therapeutic process of mapping is best guided by an individual who is in a ventral vagal state, as this is essential for creating a safe space for exploring sympathetic and dorsal vagal states (Dana 2018). Group members can use the maps to create a shared understanding that fosters better communication among them. By identifying and tracking their autonomic responses, members can begin their journey toward optimal mental health and well-being and encourage the same in others. In this way, members coregulate, and this shared experience of befriending is vital for encouraging members of the group to support one another in order to safely shift among the autonomic states.

Personal Profile Map

This map illustrates the polyvagal ladder, providing a structure for an individual to explore and document their autonomic experiences in terms of both their emotional and

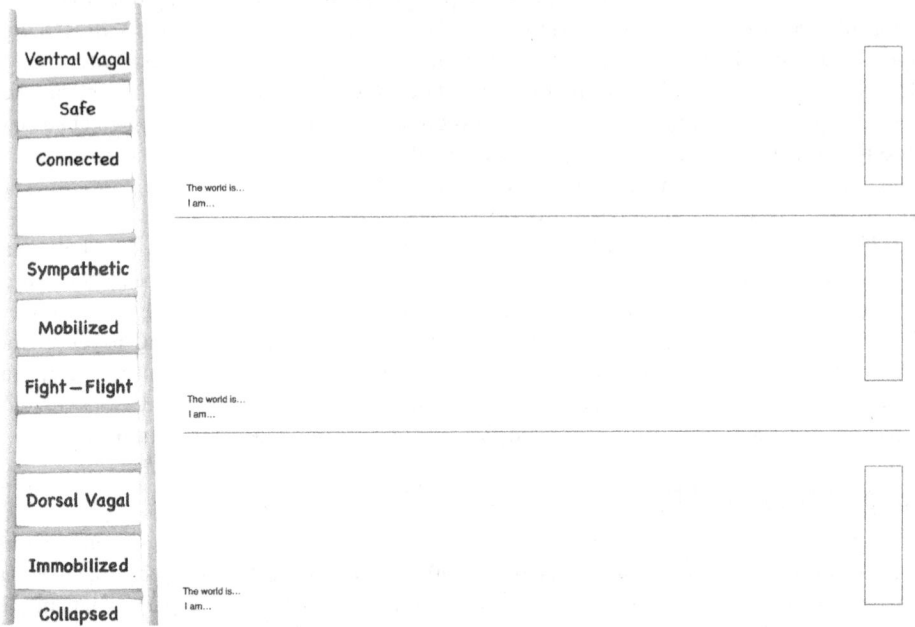

Figure 2.1 Personal Profile Map. (Source: Dana 2018.)

physiological responses. Exploring and navigating the polyvagal ladder can enhance one's overall well-being by fostering an awareness of the importance of the ventral vagal state as the desired and regulated state of connection and safety.

The map is completed by providing a printed copy to each individual; they are encouraged to use markers of different colors to fill it out. As discussed in Chapter 1, each person is invited to describe how the world seems to them in each state and how they perceive themselves. The empty boxes on the right are available if they wish to label each state with their own unique word. Some individuals prefer to use a specific color to represent each state and are invited to do so, if they wish, simply writing their responses in the corresponding color. After completing the map, they then are invited to explore the following reflection questions.

Questions for Reflection

- **"Where am I on my map?"** This question encourages the individual to reflect on their current autonomic state and become aware of their position on the autonomic hierarchy.
- **"What color am I drawn to as I prepare to map sympathetic (danger), dorsal vagal (immobilization), and ventral vagal (socialization/safety)?"** This question prompts the individual to consider the autonomic cues, even in their choice of marker colors.

Glimmers and Triggers Map

The objective of this map is to identify the factors that trigger shifts in one's autonomic states and recognize cues of danger ("triggers") that activate their sympathetic or dorsal

Triggers and Glimmers Map

Figure 2.2 The Glimmers and Triggers Map. (Source: Dana, 2018.)

vagal responses, as well as cues of safety ("glimmers") that align with health, growth, and restoration within the ventral vagal state. Recognizing the triggers for this state helps the individual gain insight into the sources of their autonomic dysregulation. This awareness allows them to proactively address and manage these triggers, potentially reducing the frequency and intensity of sympathetic and dorsal vagal responses.

Questions for Reflection

- **"What brought me here?"** This question is central to the Triggers and Glimmers Map, because it encourages group members to identify and share the personal triggers that shift them between autonomic states.
- **"What situations or events trigger my feelings of disconnection and shutdown (dorsal vagal)?"** This question is relevant because it encourages the individual to pinpoint specific circumstances or experiences that lead to feelings of isolation, withdrawal, and helplessness.
- **"When do I notice the sympathetic nervous system being activated?"** and **"What makes me feel disrespected or overwhelmed?"** These questions encourage the individual to be more aware of the circumstances that lead to fight-or-flight responses.
- **"What specific events or interactions make me feel seen and safe, bringing about a sense of ventral vagal regulation?"** This question prompts the individual to focus on positive experiences associated with the ventral vagal state, such as feelings of connection, safety, and well-being.

Regulating Resources Map

The Regulating Resources Map offers guidance for creating an action plan for enhancing social engagement and reducing shifts toward the sympathetic and dorsal vagal states. This tool helps the individual to develop self-awareness of their autonomic states and understand how to build a toolbox of strategies for moving from states of dysregulation toward the ventral vagal state of connection and well-being. The map includes one column for activities the individual can do on their own and one for activities they can do with others to improve their resilience.

Questions for Reflection

- **"How do I find my way to ventral vagal regulation?"** This question is pertinent to the Regulating Resources Map. It guides the individual in discovering the resources they need to return to the state of ventral vagal regulation.
- **"What moves me out of dorsal vagal or sympathetic dysregulation?"** Here, the individual identifies actions or strategies that can be used with others to move away from dorsal vagal or sympathetic states, such as seeking support or connecting with trusted individuals.
- **"What helps me stay in the ventral vagal state of connection and well-being?"** The individual lists activities and practices they can use to maintain a state of ventral vagal regulation. This may include mindfulness techniques, relaxation exercises, or any

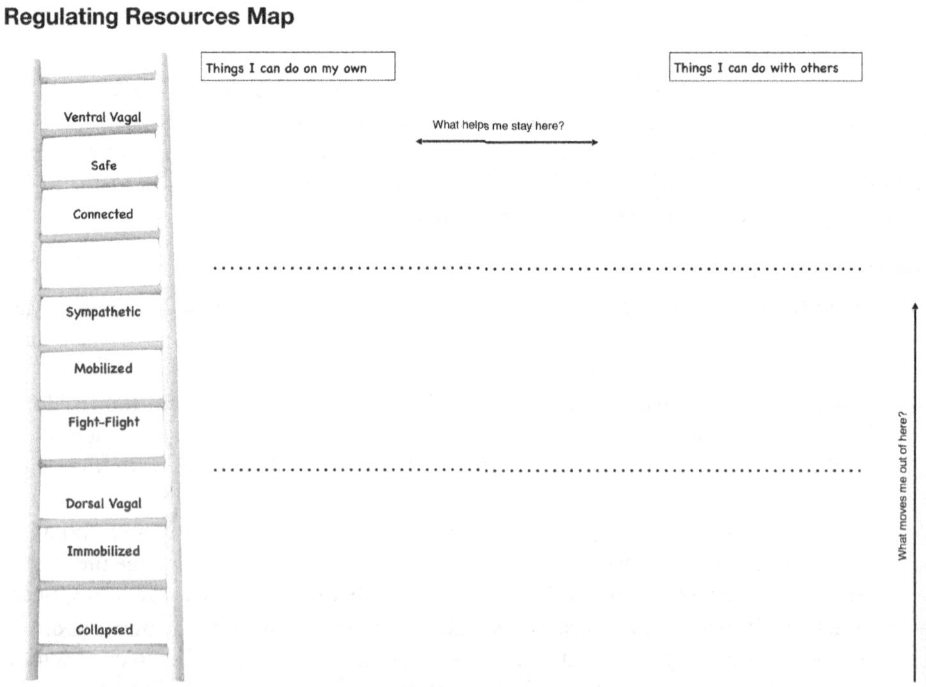

Figure 2.3 The Regulating Resources Map. (Source: Dana, 2018.)

self-soothing activities that contribute to their well-being, including the regulation exercises included in this book.

> **Case Study 2.1: Solving the Scenario**
>
> Once the clinic staff understood the basics of the PVT, they met as a group to learn how to use the ANS mapping tools to identify their autonomic states and brainstorm strategies for upregulating. Dr. Jennings initiated the process by introducing the Personal Profile Map, encouraging group members to reflect on their current autonomic state.
>
> The Personal Profile Map became a structured tool for exploring emotional and physiological responses, fostering coregulation within the group. Questions such as "Where am I on my map?" prompted self-reflection, positioning individuals on the autonomic hierarchy.
>
> To delve deeper, the Glimmers and Triggers Map was used to identify factors triggering shifts in autonomic states. Guided by questions like "What situations trigger feelings of disconnection (dorsal vagal)?," the group members pinpointed specific circumstances leading to withdrawal. Recognizing SNS activations helped them understand their stress responses, aiding in proactive management.
>
> The Regulating Resources Map was instrumental in creating an action plan. Dr. Jennings guided the group in identifying actions for moving away from dysregulated states and maintaining the ventral vagal state. This personalized toolbox encompassed both collaborative strategies with others and self-regulation activities.
>
> Dr. Jennings's holistic approach, guided by the PVT, not only addressed the challenges posed by the cognitive psychology paradigm but also empowered her team to provide more comprehensive care tailored to patient needs through the use of these tools.

Step 3: Nurture Self-Regulation Skills

The third step involves the cultivation of self-regulation skills. Polyvagal-informed interventions encourage individuals to nurture their ability to consciously regulate their ANS responses through different approaches. The most effective self-regulation strategies revolve around executive functions (goal-setting and self-monitoring), cognition (self-appraisal and self-efficacy), and responding to internal and external emotional stressors (inhibition, control, and expression) (Menefee et al. 2022).

The journey of emotional development is a process that extends across one's lifespan. According to research in the field of emotional development, there is a strong correlation between the neurobiological factors and the environmental factors that shape one's emotional regulation skills. Emotional regulation plays a vital role as people navigate their psychosocial environment since their capacity for emotional regulation is closely linked to the development of healthy self-esteem and a sense of self-efficacy. Hence, emotional regulation can strengthen a person's ability to adjust within their surrounding social environments.

Interventions that promote emotional regulation include acceptance and commitment therapy (ACT), dialectical behavior therapy (DBT), and mindfulness: ACT focuses on encouraging an individual to accept inevitable events and define goals for their respective values, while DBT is a cognitive-behavioral intervention for those with emotional dysregulation conditions, such as borderline personality disorder (Menefee et al. 2022). These self-regulation skills can empower an individual to actively take measures to manage stress, anxiety, and emotional dysregulation, all of which are major causes of undesired changes in the ANS.

In comparison, mindfulness is a straightforward approach to strengthening emotional regulation through sensory sensations. Mindfulness techniques focus on moment-to-moment awareness by enhancing how a person consciously registers occurring events and experiences. Evidence-based mindfulness techniques include yoga, meditation, and body scan exercises.

Over the past two decades, significant research has been published regarding the importance of mindfulness-based interventions for improving patients' physical and mental health outcomes. These techniques have demonstrated positive results in terms of mitigating depression and improving overall well-being and quality of life. If a person views the mind as a network that supports the flow of information between the body, brain, and relationships, it is possible to understand the central role in regulating how information is processed. With that said, mindfulness has become a popular intervention for strengthening the synergy between the body and the mind (Lucas et al. 2021). This relationship is illustrated in Figure 2.4.

Other evidence-based regulation strategies involve breathing techniques, eye and body movement, orienting attention, vocalization, and grounding meditation. Foremost, breathing techniques provide individuals with appropriate stimuli for regulating their psychological state. Fundamentally, breathing and emotions are considered bidirectional stimuli. As a result, slow breathing can increase the activity of the VVC, thereby enhancing cognition (Brown and Gerbarg 2012). This explains why slow breathing is often used as a strategy for tackling emotional and psychological events. An example is the 4–7–8 breathing exercise. In this exercise, the individual inhales for 4 seconds, holds their breath for 7 seconds, and exhales slowly for 8 seconds. This and other variations of breathing techniques can easily be incorporated in a healthcare setting to strengthen one's ability to regulate.

Another popular regulation intervention involves eye and body movements. Stable facial expressions, body movements, and eye gaze can serve as indicators of safety, contributing to the regulation of a person's autonomic response. According to Dana (2020), the presence of these features usually serves as an indicator of safety, whereas the absence of these signals often indicates danger.

Alternatively, orienting attention is an innovative approach for activating the social engagement system. Orienting attention describes a person's capacity to focus and engage with their surroundings. In reality, changes in a person's attention can significantly affect their consequent behaviors and actions. For that reason, concentration

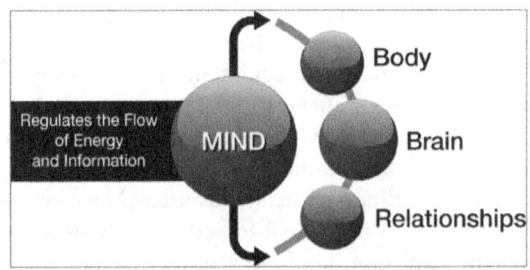

Figure 2.4 Using mindfulness to strengthen the synergy between the body, brain, and relationships. (Source: Lucas et al. 2021.)

has been deemed an effective approach for mediating a person's responses in accordance with their surroundings.

With regard to vocalization, this technique involves the use of one's vocal cords to strengthen one's inclination toward the socialization state. Reliable research demonstrates that autonomic regulation is deeply connected to listening, vocalization, and other key auditory processes (Porges 2022). Therefore, healthcare leaders can use vocalization to create a conducive work environment that promotes social engagement.

Last, grounding meditation is a well-known approach for improving one's mental, emotional, and psychological responses. Meditation is a relatively broad topic because it can involve simple activities, such as sitting, or handling complex approaches for strengthening the connection between the mind and the body. From Dana's (2020) perspective, practices such as autonomic navigation meditation have been explicitly designed to support patients in anchoring themselves in the socialization state and safely transitioning from the mobilization and immobilization states. Alternatively, guided meditation occurs when an instructor instructs the client to participate in appropriate visualization and calming exercises. Meditation creates a heightened sense of safety through guided imagery and positive feedback.

> **Case Study 2.2: Integrating PVT-Informed Approaches**
>
> Dr. Jennings is keenly aware of the increasing complexities associated with fear, stress, and anxiety among patients seeking mental health support. After teaching her staff about the PVT and how to map the ANS, she underscores the significance of fostering self-regulation skills within her team to address these challenges effectively.
>
> Recognizing emotional regulation as a pivotal aspect of mental well-being, she introduces interventions such as ACT and DBT. This recommendation involves seamlessly integrating the PVT into clinical practice, so she needs to highlight for her staff the intricate connection between the body and the mind. In addition, the introduction of mindfulness, meditation, and other self-regulation techniques can strengthen the relationship between one's body and mind, allowing one to be more receptive to social interactions and cues of safety.
>
> Through these recommendations, she will be able to empower her workers to provide more holistic care. The emphasis extends beyond mere adaptation of existing therapeutic practices; it includes optimizing the intervention to elevate the patients' responses to fear and cues of safety. By fostering an understanding of one's physical state and utilizing suitable self-regulation methods, everyone can enhance their overall emotional health and fortitude when confronting stressors.

Step 4: Strengthen Interoception

Although interoception is closely aligned with the ability to self-regulate, it focuses primarily on illuminating the communication between the body and the mind. A person's awareness of their bodily responses can play a vital role in allowing them to identify their root causes and interpret their meanings. Correspondingly, interoception provides a continuous stream of information about the body's internal state, helping individuals gauge their physiological well-being (Price and Hooven 2018). It allows them to recognize bodily signals associated with specific emotions, such as the fluttering heart of anxiety or the warmth of contentment, thereby enhancing emotional intelligence. For that reason, interoception is usually considered a blueprint for emotional regulation (Price and Hooven 2018).

Interoceptive awareness can optimize a person's response to emotional cues, thereby improving how one interprets and copes with stressful events. This heightened bodily awareness fosters a profound connection between the person and their own body, enhancing their capacity for self-care and emotional regulation. Overall, interoceptive awareness is a crucial step for strengthening the regulation of ANS responses when one is exposed to a perceived threat.

The PVT prompts healthcare professionals to consider how interoceptive dysfunctions may contribute to various mental health conditions. For instance, mood and anxiety disorders may arise when a person struggles to predict and manage their interoceptive states effectively (Khalsa et al. 2018). However, it's essential to understand whether these issues stem from sensory input, central processing in the brain, temperament, or metacognition (awareness of one's own thought processes). Beyond these, conditions such as PTSD and somatic symptom disorders are likely influenced by interoceptive dysregulation.

Changes or irregularities in interoceptive processes could serve as signs that something is amiss in the body, making it conceivable to use these measures as a way to detect diseases or health conditions earlier and with more accuracy. Correspondingly, various other disorders, including chronic pain, Tourette syndrome, borderline personality disorder, OCD, autism spectrum disorder, and functional developmental disorders, show overlaps with interoceptive symptoms (Khalsa et al. 2018). Thus, the PVT encourages a comprehensive exploration of how interoception impacts mental health and emotional well-being based on these conditions.

Interoception Guidance Exercise

With interoception being so important in our protective self-regulation responses and nervous system efforts to predict danger, it is imperative to teach interoception to others (staff and patients) as well as to strengthen it in ourselves.

There is no "right" way to experience a sensation. Some people will feel more simple and direct sensations while others have a wide and more nuanced descriptive range. Any sensation can be helpful. Generally, noticing some sensation leads to the ability to recognize more variations. Individuals should not be discouraged if interoception is simple or less available. Just like other acquired skills, this sense should start to emerge with practice.

> **Note:** Not everyone will be able to feel or identify their internal sensations. Those who are neurodivergent may not be wired to access internal sensations. In some cases, people who have experienced trauma have difficulty accessing internal sensations more immediately as a result of the necessary dissociation they experienced. Moreover, people who feel they have been judged or attacked for their identities might have less access to internal sensation at first. For others, it may be that they have never practiced feeling internal sensations. It's a new skill that can take time to learn.

1. Ensure that the environment is as comfortable as possible, and that it is not too dark or overly lit.
2. Invite others to stand, sit, or lie on the floor and take a moment to settle.
3. Ask them to notice where their body makes contact with the floor or furniture and to notice the sense of support and connection.
4. Invite them to either close their eyes or keep them open, whichever they prefer.
5. Explain the concept of interoception.
6. Review this list of basic paired opposite sensations:

- Electric/Smooth
- Heavy/Light
- Open/Stiff
- Scratchy/Smooth
- Soft/Hard
- Still/Flow
- Tight/Relaxed
- Warm/Cool

7. Ask "Can you feel one part of the body that is more (state a sensation) and one that is more (state an opposite sensation)"? Advise them to simply note what they observe to themselves. Allow about 30 seconds to 1 minute to observe.
8. Encourage the person to use any words or descriptors that they prefer if they notice an internal sensation that doesn't fall in line with the script. With practice, this may happen naturally.

Note: Sometimes internal sensations are physiological and attached to polyvagal states, and other times they are more emotional. We don't often admit to emotions in the workplace, but we are influenced by them. Fostering more positive emotional states at work and with those around us improves our quality of life and job satisfaction.

Potential Descriptors of Internal Sensations

Blobby	Fluffy	Nothing	Trembling
Buzzy	Gentle	Numb	Vibration
Disconnected	Goosebumps	Open	Void
Dry	Hard	Rigid	Warmth
Electric	Heat	Shaky	Wooden
Empty	Icy	Sludgy	Woolly
Energy	Immobile	Soft	Zappy
Flat	Insubstantial	Stuck	
Floaty	Light	Tight	
Flow	Metallic	Tingling	

Case Study 2.3: Building Interoception and Teaching the World

After teaching the basic PVT concepts and educating workers about self-regulation with the ANS mapping tools, Dr. Jennings's next step is helping the staff strengthen their own interoception, so they in turn can do the same with their patients.

Strengthening interoception involves fostering a deep understanding of the communication between the body and mind. By promoting interoceptive awareness, individuals can better interpret bodily signals associated with specific emotions. This heightened emotional intelligence enables patients like Fred Johnson (see "Case Study 2.5: Utilizing New Strategies") to recognize and understand their emotional states, facilitating more accurate self-assessment.

Dr. Jennings and her team can use this perspective to explore how difficulties in predicting and managing interoceptive states might contribute to mood and anxiety disorders. This comprehensive understanding enables a more targeted and nuanced approach to mental healthcare.

Step 5: Incorporate Polyvagal-Informed Interventions

A wide variety of polyvagal-informed interventions can be used in both individual and group settings. By customizing interventions based on the patient's preferences, experiences, and challenges, healthcare professionals can maximize the effectiveness of the treatment, leading to improved outcomes. These individual interventions include SE, eye movement desensitization and reprocessing (EMDR), trauma-informed yoga, acupuncture, aromatherapy, light therapy, sound therapy, and bodywork. Let's take a look at each.

SE

Somatic experiencing (SE) is a registered body-oriented therapeutic approach focused on treating posttraumatic symptoms by changing the way individuals perceive and respond to the bodily sensations associated with traumatic experiences. The practice is often regarded as a "bottom-up" approach because it is based on the idea that posttraumatic stress symptoms stem from a continuous overreaction of the innate stress response system (Kuhfuß et al. 2021).

In SE, clients are guided to shift their attention to internal bodily sensations, such as visceral (interoception) and musculoskeletal (proprioception and kinaesthesis) awareness, instead of primarily concentrating on cognitive or emotional aspects. This differs notably from cognitive-behavioral therapy, which primarily addresses cognitive and emotional experiences linked to trauma.

From there onward, clients gradually reduce the heightened arousal associated with trauma through downregulation or upregulation of the nervous system, as well as through movements associated with success in primitive fight-or-flight or mastery responses. In essence, the nervous system plays out a different successful outcome, much like when an athlete uses visualization and subtle movement to train the brain. They can also utilize internal and external resources, such as identifying body parts or memories associated with positive feelings.

In addition, it is crucial to highlight that SE avoids forcing clients to directly relive traumatic memories; instead, it encourages them to address the memories indirectly and gradually. This approach allows for the design of interventions that strengthen the person's interoceptive experiences and counteract their feelings of helplessness. Somatic experiencing's connection to the PVT lies in its emphasis on regulating physiological responses, particularly the role of interoception and bodily sensations in influencing emotional states.

EMDR

Eye movement desensitization and reprocessing (EMDR) is a validated psychotherapy method for treating psychological trauma and the consequences of negative life experiences. The intervention can provide relief from unprocessed memories associated with those experiences. It can be applied to a wide range of medical and psychological issues affecting both patients and their families.

The therapy comprises eight distinct phases: history-taking, educating and training appropriate clients on the technique, assessment of processing targets, desensitization of traumatic experiences, installation of positive cognitive networks, body scanning for residual disturbances, closure of EMDR sessions, and reassessment to maintain therapeutic outcomes (Shapiro 2014).

In relation to the PVT, EMDR focuses on the therapy's ability to address the physiological and psychological responses to trauma. By targeting and processing distressing memories, EMDR can help rewire the patient's ANS, thereby improving self-regulation and reducing the body's heightened stress responses (Shapiro 2014). Overall, the intervention can lead to a drastic improvement in a patient's mental and physical well-being.

Trauma-Informed Yoga

Trauma-informed yoga is a mindful approach to yoga that considers the specific needs and experiences of individuals who have suffered trauma. In this therapy, the focus is on developing mindfulness and enhancing one's connection to the body and brain through captivating yoga postures, breathing techniques, and relaxation methods that are tailored to the individual's comfort and pace (West et al. 2017).

Existing research on trauma interventions highlights that traditional interventions often fail to fully address the patient's symptoms. Trauma-informed yoga emerged as a promising technique for strengthening one's physical and mental state. Through the practice, it is possible to help individuals with a history of trauma to build interoceptive awareness and develop emotional regulation skills (West et al. 2017). Patients who rely on this technique can comprehend how physiological states influence emotional well-being and behavior. Additionally, they can learn to regulate their ANS, thereby reducing the negative emotional impacts associated with trauma. Although trauma-informed yoga has similar characteristics to traditional yoga, it differs due to its inherent focus on alleviating mental health problems such as stress and anxiety.

Acupuncture

Acupuncture is a therapeutic technique that involves the insertion of thin needles into specific points on the body to promote healing and alleviate various health conditions. In most cases, it is employed as an alternative to long-term medication due to its perceived fewer side effects and good tolerance. In current times, acupuncture is recognized as an effective complementary and alternative therapy that can target various mental disorders, such as anxiety disorders, panic disorders, phobias, and social anxiety disorders (Yang et al. 2021).

The technique works by stimulating specific points on the body, which are believed to influence the flow of energy (qi) and the body's overall balance. This stimulation is thought to trigger natural healing responses, reduce pain, and alleviate symptoms associated with a wide range of health issues. Acupuncture's potential impact on a patient's mental health largely revolves around the PVT's principles of interoception and emotional regulation.

Aromatherapy

Emerging research on aromatherapy – the therapeutic use of essential oils – reveals that certain smells can trigger unique autonomic responses, which clearly aligns this ancient practice with the PVT (Langley-Brady et al. 2023). For instance, pungent and sour smells tend to induce the mobilization and immobilization states. For example, when a person smells smoke, they become more susceptible to the flight-or-fight response because smoke is often associated with fire. Comparatively, sweet smells can arouse positive memories, and other scents, such as lavender, can have an overall calming effect.

Aromatherapy offers a convenient approach for enhancing mood and emotional regulation. In fact, it is considered one of the leading complementary and alternative medicines (CAM), having been used in a wide diversity of cultures and healthcare settings (Van der Watt and Janca 2008). Through the lens of psychophysiology, aromatherapy helps modulate a person's optimal state of arousal and positive emotional valence. Operating through a simple process, the essential oil molecules are usually inhaled through the mouth and nose, allowing them to reach the brain. Thereafter, the PNS is activated, prompting stress relief.

Several essential oils have gained significant attention due to their ability to strengthen mental well-being and promote relaxation, including lavender, bergamot, and marjoram (Ke et al. 2022). In the healthcare environment, where stress is common, diffusing certain stress-relieving essential oils can contribute to a more relaxed atmosphere and improved employee well-being.

While conventional medicines and therapeutic interventions are used as the first-line intervention for mental health issues, emerging research highlights that non-conventional and alternative medicines can be adopted to complement evidence-based interventions or replace them (Van der Watt and Janca 2008).

One caveat is that for some patients with PTSD, certain smells can be a trigger, and many mental health facilities have a policy that precludes staff from using perfumes or colognes. Others may be sensitive to natural and synthetic chemicals. Additionally, natural essential oils, even in a diffuser, may be unpleasant or activate a shift on the polyvagal ladder to the sympathetic or dorsal vagal state. Healthcare leaders could opt to have only certain rooms and areas available for the use of scents and ensure that patients and staff have the option to exclude themselves from these areas.

Given the large number of essential oils to choose from, it can be challenging to identify scents that match someone's emotional or psychological needs. Fundamentally, different people have varying preferences, and this problem highlights the importance of exploring various aromas to improve the effectiveness of aromatherapy interventions. To achieve this goal, individuals are recommended to use evidence-based aromatherapy tools, such as the fragrance wheel (Plant Therapy 2019). The fragrance wheel categorizes the basic aromas according to specific classifications based on their scents and properties. According to Michailidou et al. (2023), the tool is commonly used by perfumers to classify fragrances according to specific olfactory groups to distinguish their similarities and differences. Figure 2.5 illustrates how the fragrance wheel categorizes the main olfactory groups. The fragrance wheel is a crucial instrument for revitalizing a person's autonomic state according to ten groups: floral, medicinal, herbal, green, earthy, food-like, mint, fruity, wood, and spice.

In addition to this research, a large number of studies have been performed on the mechanisms of infusion. For instance, the traditional approach involved the inhalation of essential oils through diffusers. This approach is relatively convenient for the office layout, where workers are separated according to their departments. However, the evolution of healthcare technology has seen the emergence of nasal inhalers that support brain-targeted nasal delivery and offer greater aromatherapy benefits. The inhalation of these essential oils

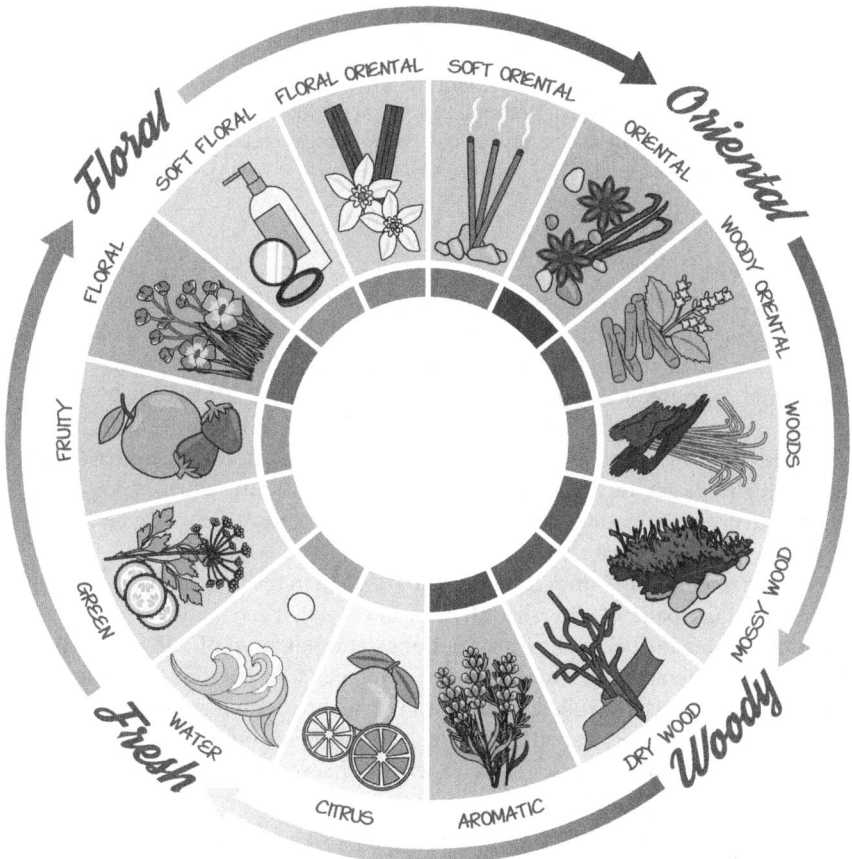

Figure 2.5 The Fragrance Wheel. (Source: MedejaJa/iStock/Getty Images Plus.)

sends signals directly to the olfactory system, thereby allowing the brain to produce specific physiological responses. This technique has demonstrated significant results in treating mood disorders (Cui et al. 2022). Considering the nervous link between the olfactory system and the brain, corporate leaders are encouraged to implement appropriate aromatherapy interventions to improve their workers' well-being and productivity.

> **Case Study 2.4: Using Aromatherapy**
>
> Aromatherapy can be used to alleviate stress and promote well-being in hospital staff and patients. Healthcare leaders could use aromatherapy as a complementary intervention for reducing stress and strengthening cues of safety. This can be achieved by installing essential

oil diffusers in patient waiting rooms, lobbies, and other areas to create a relaxing atmosphere for welcoming healthcare stakeholders. Furthermore, bedding, linen, and blankets can be infused with these oils to improve their ability to soothe, through the use of sprays or scented detergents.

In reality, most healthcare facilities tend to smell of cleaning agents and disinfectants that are designed to convey that the clinic is a sterile environment. The introduction of aromatherapy is intended to complement these initiatives by creating an appealing environment that encourages occupants to remain in the social engagement state instead of shifting to mobilization or immobilization states. With 10 family groups to choose from, Dr. White has a long list of essential oils he can use to create the desired atmosphere at Safe Haven Clinic.

Light Therapy

Light therapy, or phototherapy, is a common treatment involving exposure to a specified amount of artificial light to treat a specific mental health condition. The technique influences one's circadian rhythm, serotonin secretion, and alertness based on the duration, wavelength, and frequency of exposure to light. For example, bright light therapy (BLT) is a treatment approach that involves exposure to bright and full-spectrum light to alleviate various conditions. Initially developed to treat seasonal affective disorder (SAD), BLT has shown high efficacy in addressing numerous mental health issues, such as unipolar and bipolar depression, eating disorders, and adult attention deficit/hyperactivity disorder (ADHD) (Campbell et al. 2017).

Light has a profound impact on the visual system in the brain, which is part of the VVC. By influencing a patient's circadian rhythm and mood, it is possible to positively mold their emotional states and behaviors. Interventions stemming from BLT involve daily exposure to bright light, generally in the morning. Key parameters, such as light intensity and duration, should be carefully controlled to ensure the patient is comfortable. However, healthcare practitioners should be aware that too much intense light could activate the SNS and worsen anxiety. For example, a person who experienced severe stress from a medical procedure such as surgery may find that bright lights serve as a reminder of the intense lighting in the operating room, triggering a fear response.

Sound Therapy

Another popular technique that has gained significant traction is sound therapy. Sound therapy, often referred to as sound healing or sound meditation, is an integrative medicine technique that employs vibrational musical instruments to promote emotional and spiritual empowerment (Goldsby et al. 2022).

The survival of humanity can be largely attributed to their ability to identify cues of safety and danger from the sounds in their surroundings. According to the PVT, the ANS is innately designed to respond to specific sounds and frequencies because they influence the activation/inhibition of the ventral vagal system. As a result, low-frequency sounds can trigger the body to enter the sympathetic or dorsal vagal response because of the assumption of danger. For example, low-frequency sounds, such as the sound of thunder, are often associated with immobilization. Similarly, high-frequency and unpredictable sounds can pull a person's attention and make them more attentive to danger, such as a shrill scream that could serve as a signal of pain and danger.

"Acoustic comfort" is a term that has emerged directly due to the strong relationship between sound and the autonomic state. It describes the subjective perception of a person's acoustic environment to determine whether one achieves satisfaction. To achieve acoustic comfort, healthcare facilities need to create acoustic environments that reflect the needs and preferences of their staff and patients.

Sound therapy is often associated with audio processing, or how the nervous system processes and responds to auditory stimuli such as sounds and voices. One such example of sound therapy is the Safe and Sound Protocol (SSP). This is a patented technology that relies on PVT concepts to revolutionize mental health therapy. A series of five 60-minute recordings are played through earphones following a trained therapist's instructions and can be administered in the office or at home. The music is filtered through a patented and evidence-based algorithm that eliminates frequencies associated with cues of danger and can thus assist in regulating the ANS by infusing the brain with cues of safety. It is specifically designed to stimulate the vagus nerve and enhance the social engagement system (the ventral vagal state), aiming to promote healing and connection. Overall, it creates a safe space for integrating the brain and body to achieve long-lasting mental health benefits. Follow-up research reveals that listening to sound can decrease auditory hypersensitivity and improve emotional regulation, spontaneous speech, and behavioral organization (Porges 2021b).

The Music of Voice
Sound therapy also encompasses the "music of the voice." In essence, a person's tone and pitch can create a soothing rhythm that allows them to effectively convey their emotional state. Dana (2018) claims that *prosody* (the music of the voice) can play an important role in communicating what lies beneath the speaker's words and intent. For instance, a monotone voice that is too shrill or deep can trigger the ANS to be attentive to danger, whereas a voice with appropriate patterns tends to encourage listers to feel a safe connection.

Many human beings have an inherent ability to recognize vocal cues and determine when they are out of sync with one's emotions. This explains why most therapists alter the pitch of their voices to match their clients' emotional states and create a sense of safety. For example, some therapists repeat that "everything is okay" to lull the patient's ANS and stimulate the social engagement system to perceive safety instead of threats. Voice therapy is a commonly used approach for assist the ANS to inhibit the body from shifting to the mobilization state.

Case Study 2.5: Utilizing New Strategies

Dr. Jennings can use multiple strategies to improve Fred Johnson's mental and physical well-being.

Somatic experiencing, a body-oriented therapeutic approach, aligns with the PVT's emphasis on regulating physiological responses. It focuses on shifting attention to internal bodily sensations, promoting interoceptive experiences, and countering feelings of helplessness. Dr. Jennings can integrate SE to help Fred gradually reduce the heightened arousal associated with his anxiety by acknowledging and tolerating inner physical sensations, contributing to improved emotional regulation. For example, it could be argued that Fred's anxiety stems from hyperarousal of the nervous system to past events, which has led to his staying stuck in incomplete responses and which SE could help him resolve.

Additionally, EMDR can help the patient's physiological and psychological responses to trauma, either alone or in combination with other interventions. By targeting distressing memories, EMDR can rewire Fred's ANS, enhancing self-regulation and reducing heightened stress responses. This intervention has the potential to significantly improve Fred's mental and physical well-being.

Dr. Jennings can also use trauma-informed yoga. Trauma-informed yoga is designed to consider the specific needs of trauma survivors as well as those suffering from stress and anxiety, so it could be a valuable tool for helping Fred. It can be used alone or in combination with other approaches, depending on the person's preference. This mindful approach fosters interoceptive awareness and emotional regulation. Through tailored yoga postures and relaxation methods, Fred can develop a stronger connection to his body and enhance his capacity for self-care, aligning with the holistic approach of the PVT.

Another approach is acupuncture, which supports interoception and emotional regulation. By stimulating specific points in the body, acupuncture aims to influence the flow of energy and restore balance. This intervention can contribute to Fred's mental health by promoting natural healing responses, reducing pain, and alleviating symptoms associated with his social anxiety disorder. Acupuncture often seeks to restore a more normal balance between sympathetic and parasympathetic tone in the nervous system.

Furthermore, aromatherapy offers a complementary and natural approach to stress reduction. Dr. Jennings can introduce aromatherapy to Fred as a means of improving emotional regulation and overall well-being. The calming effects of essential oils can potentially reduce stress and anxiety, aligning with the PVT's emphasis on optimizing ANS responses.

Bright light therapy offers Dr. Jennings an opportunity to positively influence Fred's circadian rhythm and mood. By incorporating daily exposure to bright light, Dr. Jennings can explore its potential to optimize Fred's emotional states and behaviors. Careful consideration of light intensity and duration is crucial to ensure a comfortable and effective application of this intervention.

Finally, sound therapy can be integrated into Fred's mental healthcare plan to sooth him and strengthen his body–mind connection. Dr. Jennings can explore the benefits of sound therapy in reducing stress, anxiety, and depression, offering a unique approach to activating the parasympathetic branch of the ANS associated with relaxation and calm. Fred would be a good potential candidate for the SSP.

Step 6: Consider Group Interventions

While individualized treatment is crucial for providing patient-centered care, group interventions are usually more effective in terms of encouraging patients to share their experiences. These interventions can break down feelings of isolation and anxiety by promoting positive social interactions, thereby strengthening the ventral vagal state of socialization. Overall, group interventions allow patients to exercise their knowledge in real-life healthcare settings. Reliable group interventions include introducing the PVT in a group setting, mapping the ANS with worksheets, and teaching group members about self-regulation.

By fostering a sense of safety and social engagement within the group, participants can gain insights, develop coping skills, and strengthen their mental health. This approach aligns with the holistic principles of the PVT, emphasizing the crucial role of social engagement and safety in psychological well-being and recovery. When individuals within the group feel secure the VVC is activated, thereby promoting social engagement and trust.

This process is especially critical for individuals struggling with specific mental health issues, such as stress, trauma, loneliness, or stigma.

By incorporating the PVT into group interventions, practitioners can become attuned to the physiological responses of group members. The group bond is an important consideration in such settings because it represents the feelings of cohesion of the entire group (Ezhumalai et al. 2018). Techniques such as deep breathing, mindfulness, and grounding exercises can significantly assist the group members in managing their problems and develop a profound sense of safety within the group. Patients can also perform activities that offer insight into their autonomic states and propose recommendations for improving their resilience against external threats.

Group interventions are more effective than individual interventions in terms of promoting coregulation. For instance, gym-goers who attend group workouts tend to motivate each other to expand their limits, thereby encouraging each other to be more productive. In these settings, the members acknowledge that they are not alone in their struggles. Participants can learn from others who have similar or different challenges, and the variety of viewpoints can help normalize their own experiences. Furthermore, the participants can share their progress and receive encouragement from their peers. This sense of responsibility to the group can be a strong motivating factor for individuals to engage actively in the therapeutic process.

Given that most polyvagal-informed techniques focus on improving the patient's self-regulation and social engagement skills, the members can gain opportunities to practice their skills and experiment with new possibilities. Therefore, group interventions are feasible settings for implementing polyvagal-informed techniques in the group setting.

> **Case Study 2.6: Changing Lives in the Group Setting**
>
> Dr. Jennings wishes to offer patients of the clinic support in a group setting. She recognizes the importance of group interventions in fostering a sense of safety and social engagement.
>
> After training her staff, some of the therapists volunteered to incorporate their new learning and tools in a therapeutic group and quickly recruited twelve clients who suffered from anxiety to participate in weekly sessions.
>
> Accordingly, while in the group the participants normalized their experiences and learned from others who shared similar challenges. In addition, group members actively practiced polyvagal-informed techniques, experimenting with new possibilities for self-regulation and social engagement. As a result, these activities resulted in positive changes in the members' mental and social functioning. In the end, patients struggling with stress, trauma, and loneliness found a supportive community where they could interact and exchange ideas.

Step 7: Provide Cues of Safety

The final step for implementing polyvagal-informed interventions in the healthcare setting is to create a conducive environment that exudes safety. This step requires healthcare professionals to use cues of safety to promote physical and emotional safety. Cues of safety are subtle signals that are processed beneath conscious awareness (Dana 2018). It is crucial to understand that the ANS is sensitive to features of the environment. For instance, certain sounds activate ventral vagal safety, while temperature affects thermal comfort and can influence the autonomic state, positively or negatively (Dana 2018). Similarly, exposure to natural elements such as nature scenes and water promotes a parasympathetic response, thereby reducing stress and enhancing well-being.

Healthcare professionals can provide cues of safety through tone of voice, eye contact, facial expressions, nonverbal cues, and conducive interior designs. Let's review what's involved in each.

Tone of Voice

Tone of voice refers to the emotional quality and pitch used when speaking. Vocal cues related to tone of voice are linked to demonstrating the speaker's social desirability, activity, and intelligence. Among these, social desirability is usually determined when a person perceives the following elements in a person's voice: kindness, honesty, trustworthiness, and warmth (Chappuis and Grandjean 2022).

Tone of voice is a powerful tool for conveying emotions and personality traits so it can contribute significantly to feelings of safety during social interactions. For instance, a harsh or unfriendly tone of voice can cause discomfort and insecurity in others, while a warm, friendly tone can make them feel at ease, thereby fostering a sense of security and comfort in social interactions.

Eye Contact

Eye contact is a popular strategy for assessing threats and danger based on the speakers' social interactions. Similar to tone of voice, making eye contact with others is crucial for conveying a sense of safety. In this state, individuals are more likely to express themselves openly, share their thoughts and feelings, and engage in constructive social interactions. The sense of safety created by eye contact can be particularly important in group settings, where it encourages individuals to speak up and participate actively (Abi-Esber et al. 2022). In contrast, when people perceive a lack of eye contact or a hostile gaze it can trigger defensive responses, leading to feelings of threat and discomfort. In such situations, individuals are less likely to speak up or engage openly. Too much eye contact can be seen as a sign of aggression, whereas too little eye contact can be seen as avoidance. These perceptions can occur even when the intention was not to be negative or threatening.

Facial Expressions

When facial expressions convey safety, people can engage, communicate, and interact with confidence and comfort. Relaxed eyes and mouth, with a gentle smile, convey warmth and friendliness, for example. Healthcare professionals should be mindful as to how their expressions are received and make efforts to look welcoming. With practice, one can develop skill over time and be able to use a more neutral or friendly expression. That said, some people are typically more expressive and may struggle to conceal their emotions. Mindfulness exercises can help an individual learn to present a more neutral expression. By promoting a state of calm and social engagement, nonthreatening facial expressions serve as cues for safety, fostering an environment wherein people feel secure and free to express themselves.

The meaning of a facial expression can change based on what we learn about the situation (Guarnera et al. 2015). For example, a smile is traditionally associated with happiness, but that same smile can be threatening on a dangerous person's face. This adaptability to interpret facial expressions based upon available information is significant in our understanding of how humans process cues of safety and threat.

The underlying relationship between facial expressions and human emotions has been a major topic of research for many decades. Various charts depicting different facial expressions and the emotional state they signify are common in child/adolescent behavioral health clinics, helping children better understand their own emotional state as well as that of others. This, however, doesn't include micro expressions (quick, involuntary expressions of an emotion), which can lead to a changing landscape of facial expressions to interpret. Considering the large number facial expressions, it can be relatively difficult for a person to understand the emotional or psychological significance of each expression (LoBue, Baker and Thrasher 2017). Nevertheless, understanding how to use facial expressions as cues of safety is essential for bolstering interpersonal communication.

If you want to practice softening your face, look in a mirror, or sit or stand in a private space, and experiment with yawning, squinting, and opening your eyes, scrunching and relaxing your mouth, and raising and lowering your forehead. If you are using a mirror, make a facial expression that displays happiness, then friendliness, then anger, then fear, and see how that may or may not cause different sensations within your body, triggering some interoception. You can do this for just a minute or two and then try to relax the muscles around your eyes, forehead, temples, mouth, and cheeks before interacting with others.

Body Language and Gestures

Mastering communication is more than just words; it's about decoding the unspoken. Aside from facial expressions, other nonverbal cues can also provide valuable information about a person's thoughts and emotions, through body language and gestures. This explains why most individuals use nonverbal cues to complement verbal communication. Instead of using words to communicate with others, a simple smile or a raised eyebrow can convey a crucial message or interpretation to someone else. Therefore, healthcare professionals need to be savvy in their use of nonverbal communication cues to create an environment that exudes safety.

There are many resources available to help coach around nonverbal communication skills. Examples include the use of appropriate eye contact, an open posture, smiling and keeping a relaxed facial expression when congruent with the situation (you may want to not smile if someone is distraught or ashamed, for example), and learning skills to mirror the other person (which lets them know you are paying attention). Additionally, hand gestures, arm movements, and even providing respectful personal space can be powerful.

Physical Proximity

The physical proximity – that is, the closeness or distance – between two or more conversing individuals can speak volumes about their levels of trust and perceptions of safety. In some cultures, standing too close can be a sign of threat or intimidation, whereas in others standing too far away is seen as disrespectful. This also varies from individual to individual, based on each person's internal boundary map; notice how some people prefer to stand closer to you whereas others keep more of a distance. For the healthcare professional, one could simply ask the patient or fellow worker what their preference is. Otherwise, observe the other person's body language to ascertain whether you need to close in or back away a bit.

Physical proximity can convey various messages and may have a profound impact on the dynamics of a given situation. For instance, whether the speakers stand close enough to share a secret or maintain a respectful distance, they communicate various messages that can transform the atmosphere of any given situation.

Being aware of the silent language of physical proximity is a skill that can enhance an individual's professional relationships. Developing an understanding of cultural differences is also paramount, and it may be safest to assume more distance is better, until you have sufficient time to assess the situation. Additionally, holding a slightly oblique stance may be less threatening, as it avoids full frontal confrontation.

Demeanor and Energy Levels

Demeanor and energy levels pertain to a person's overall attitude and vitality. These nonverbal aspects of behavior reveal whether someone is calm, excited, anxious, or relaxed, significantly impacting the atmosphere of a conversation. For instance, slouched shoulders and a monotonous voice may indicate a lack of enthusiasm, while a lively disposition with animated gestures signals high energy and engagement. These cues significantly impact the overall quality of communication, helping individuals understand each other's emotional states and adapt their responses accordingly.

It is generally recommended that your nervous system state partially matches the patient's. For example, if they are agitated and irritable, you would show some ventral vagal plus friendly sympathetic energy, rather than trying to portray a relaxed, low-energy state, to avoid further irritating them. When we match the state of others with friendly ventral vagal energy, we let them know that we see them and are there with them. This provides important cues of safety.

Language of Design

The language of design is an innovative strategy for conveying specific messages or safety cues. In this context, it involves the use of architectural and environmental features to appeal to viewers and create feelings of safety and comfort within them. This includes considering lighting, color schemes, building layouts and views, furniture, and sound mitigation. One can easily imagine how a facility that is too harsh or bright, with many hard surfaces, will not seem as warm or calming as one that has windows with pleasant views that allow natural light. As a result, the language of design can impact how individuals perceive and experience their surroundings. This topic is covered in more detail in Chapter 6.

> **Case Study 2.7: Using Nonverbal Cues of Safety**
>
> By incorporating cues of safety aligned with the passive pathways of the ANS, Dr. Jennings aims to enhance Fred's social engagement, resilience, and overall decision-making.
>
> Dr. Jennings and her team employ a warm and friendly tone of voice as a foundational element in their interactions with Fred. This deliberate choice is rooted in their understanding of the profound connection between tone and key social attributes such as desirability, kindness, honesty, and trustworthiness. The intentional use of a warm tone creates a secure space where effective communication and emotional expression can flourish, contributing significantly to Fred's overall well-being.

Eye contact is also crucial. Within group sessions and individual interactions, Dr. Jennings emphasizes the importance of positive and affirming eye contact. Recognizing that eye contact serves as a nonverbal bridge to connection, the team ensures its consistent application to make Fred and other patients feel seen and acknowledged. This practice is particularly impactful in group settings, where the shared acknowledgment through eye contact enhances the overall sense of safety.

The team's commitment to cultivating an environment of safety can also be seen in the careful education of the workers about their facial expressions. By utilizing facial expressions that convey safety and trust, as described previously, they create a space wherein Fred feels secure to engage, communicate openly, and share his thoughts and feelings. As part of their training, the healthcare workers can practice skills that allow them to present as calm and neutral, even if they feel differently. The core of this is to have them learn the basic regulation skills described earlier, to shift their state from dorsal vagal or sympathetic to a more ventral vagal one. When calmer and more aware of their own internal interoception and emotions, it becomes easier to modify how they present to the external world. This intentional use of facial expressions serves as a powerful means of nonverbal communication, enriching the therapeutic environment.

Nonverbal cues are as essential as verbal ones. Understanding the significance of nonverbal communication, Dr. Jennings and her team adeptly decode Fred's unspoken messages, as conveyed through his body language and gestures. These nonverbal cues, meticulously synchronized with verbal communication, provide additional layers of information for a deeper understanding of Fred's emotions and needs. By being attuned to these subtleties, the team is able to provide individualized support to Fred, thereby creating a sense of safety within the healthcare setting.

Dr. Jennings can also use the language of physical proximity to impact the dynamics of the patient's interactions. Whether offering support by standing close or allowing space for comfort, the team's deliberate management of physical proximity contributes to an atmosphere that aligns with Fred's preferred comfort level. This heightened awareness ensures that the physical environment respects and accommodates Fred's needs.

Demeanor and energy levels can also influence feelings of safety. The demeanor and energy levels maintained by Dr. Jennings and her team need to be carefully altered to create a positive and welcoming atmosphere, by using regulation skills and a mindful approach to how they both feel and present to the external world. Through their engagement and lively disposition, they contribute to an environment that is professionally conducive and inviting. This positive atmosphere will strengthen Fred's overall sense of safety and create a therapeutic setting where he feels supported and encouraged.

The physical environment within the clinic should enhance feelings of safety and comfort for both staff and patients. Dr. Jennings intentionally chose architectural and environmental features to create a space that is based on established guidance around lighting, color, and textures to provide cues of safety. This strategic design not only contributes to a positive perception of the surroundings but also actively promotes an environment wherein Fred and other patients feel at ease.

Combining the Concepts in the Healthcare Setting

Let's explore how to use the PVT in relationship to your interactions with others in the healthcare setting. Using the tools we have shared with you thus far, it is essential to first check your own state before interacting with others and take steps to regulate your ANS.

(These tools are taught in more detail in our NeuroConsulting workshops; see the Conclusion for more information on scheduling a workshop.)

Polyvagal Promotions Protocol

Once you have learned and practiced the regulation skills detailed in Chapter 1 and implemented the nonverbal communication skills covered in this chapter, the next stage is to accurately observe the other person and help them to return to a more ventral vagal state of social engagement. We have developed the following protocol to outline the steps you can take to try to achieve this. Be aware that you will not be successful every time, and if the other person is too agitated or shut down you may need to leave the situation and revisit it at another time. Of course, if there is an imminent danger issue, this needs to be dealt with according to your organization's policies and procedures.

There are three stages and two approaches in this protocol. The stages are (1) Stay, (2) Change, and (3) Challenge. The approaches are "comments" and "activities." Each stage covers all three ANS states, with comments and activities for each. In comments, we give examples of things you might say and the activities that invite action or mobilization.

Stay Comments

You first interpret the polyvagal state of your patient. Your questions will match the state you identify. Stay where they are for now, meeting the patient in their dominant polyvagal state. Don't change or challenge them as to where they are on the polyvagal ladder; simply hold that reflection for a time. This is important because when people feel met and accurately reflected, they may be able to better take in relational cues of safety. The following are examples of comments you could make to acknowledge them in each of the three states on the polyvagal ladder.

Ventral Vagal

- It's nice to see you today. Are those new glasses? (Patient is looking at you.)
- I really hear what you're saying. (Middle ear tuning into the sound of the patient's voice while the patient is explaining something.)
- Thank you for listening. (Middle ear, they are tuning into you.)
- It's good to laugh with you. You've got a great sense of humor. (Emotional mirroring of positive state.)
- I value connection too. (If the patient is expressing a desire for someone to help them and listen to them, engaging our need for connection.)

SNS

- That sounds so challenging. I hear all the things you've done to try to make it better. (You can specifically list the actions the person has taken to try to protect or advocate for themselves or loved ones, such as "You really spoke up"; "You set a clear boundary"; "You knew your limits and when to step away.")
- Does it feel better to talk about all of it even though it's a lot?
- I see/hear how mobilized you are around this.
- I hear how angry you are. It must feel so frustrating, irritating, and unfair.

Dorsal Vagal

- I hear how exhausted you are.
- This is so heavy.
- You sound pretty stuck. I hear how difficult it is.
- It's like you're wanting to disappear. That sounds like a natural reaction to an overwhelming situation/or to all the challenges you've faced and are trying to overcome.

Change Comments

The next stage takes note of the patient's polyvagal state, but now the idea is to try to shift it upward, or at least slightly toward more regulation. These comments gently invite a small but important change. You can also notice activities that a client is doing that might be naturally aligning with a changing state.

SNS

- What a busy time! This is where the comfy new office chairs come in handy. What do you think of them?
- That all seems super stressful, and you've been going and going. I am glad we can have this meeting so you can have some time to focus on your needs. Or I am glad we can have this meeting to slow things down that we can figure out some new directions.
- Hearing all the things you're managing it's no wonder you've been in hyperdrive and feeling anxious. Let's take some time to recognize everything you do for the company, and also figure out how to get you a sense of a steadier pace, just like right now – we have plenty of time.

Dorsal Vagal

- I get a sense that you feel you can't handle another thing. You are handling being at this meeting, and that is something. Or you're handling talking to me. Let's take it step by step.
- I hear how depressed you've been. Let's look at what is overwhelming you, but also if there are a few things you're doing that are better for you. Are there small things in the office or that you're doing that pull you out a little bit? Why do you think those things are helpful?
- If you're thinking that life isn't worth living, I learned that might be like a freeze response. I know some good therapists who partner with our company in polyvagal theory who you could see. I am glad you told me, that you're talking to people so you're not alone. Can I get you some names for a referral? And who else can you talk to?

Challenge Comments

These comments take note of a person's polyvagal state and challenge them to shift to a more desirable state. For example, those in sympathetic states need more calming from the parasympathetic VVC, and those in dorsal vagal states need more SNS activation to pull them out of immobilization. Here are several examples:

SNS

- That all seems stressful. I'm worried about you. What could you do to reduce some stress? If you can't do less, can you shift the pace or the intensity that you're working from? Sometimes it's the internal state more than the stress of a task itself.

- When I am stressed like that I try to do some regulation. I move my attention to my legs. Or I notice if there is a sensation where I don't feel stressed. Sometimes I just look at something and really enjoy it without complications. Not on the phone – in real life. It tells us that nothing bad is actually happening right now in this moment. The brain can take a break from overload and sometimes we feel a little lighter. Collecting moments of "okayness" throughout the day helps me interrupt chronic stress.
- You haven't slowed down since you've arrived. Let's talk about something else for a moment. I want to hear what you have to say, and your thoughts and body reactions have a strong influence on each other. You mentioned one thing that was going okay – can you tell me more about that first? How were you able to make that a success?

Dorsal Vagal

- I feel the devastation too. Such a burden you're under. That weight could crush a person, but here you are. You keep showing up; something is moving you forward even if you can't sense it. Do you see the silver lining there in the cloud?
- It's so hard. And you're stuck. But take a minute to see that you're looking at me. You're looking for a solution here and in yourself. Notice your inner sensations and the room around you, paying attention to both inside and outside of yourself. You wouldn't be here if there wasn't any hope.
- Sometimes we all feel down, and it doesn't seem like anything will help. What can you do to mobilize yourself out of this? Is there anything that *is* working, and can we build on that? Can you break up the immobilization with a little movement toward something? Let's look at a realistic goal.

Stay Activities

Ventral Vagal

- Sure, you can move your chair closer if you need to hear better or see me better. (Patient moves more into proximal contact with you, and within a comfortable range for you as well.)
- It's good to see you again too. Is there anything you'd like to tackle during your visit today?
- Let's sit and spend some time. It's good to hear how you've been doing.

SNS

- It's great you have come here. You've taken action to get help. Our survival instincts are there to protect us and ensure we get through okay.
- I know it's overwhelming right now. I bet that bouncing of your leg helps.
- Do you want to walk around the room with some of that excess charge for a minute before we continue?
- I saw that gesture with your hand a second ago – seems like you were instinctively trying to protect yourself from the situation you're talking about, or a way to keep yourself safe from the fall/accident/etc.

Dorsal Vagal

- It's fine if you want to lean back on the pillow on the couch and just let yourself feel the exhaustion.

- Let's take it slow. You don't need to rush out of here or to get your things together immediately.
- How would it be to just let yourself feel collapsed and be honest with it? You're in a heavy place – how about *not* having to fight it right now for a little while?

Change Activities

You can invite a client to do a physical movement or perform a task that will change or challenge a dominant survival state.

SNS

- That's a lot of energy you're maintaining to keep on top of everything. What happens if you slow your general movement down?
- Take a moment to look around and see if there is any urgency here you have to tend to right now?
- Let's do the same movement with more awareness in it. Does that help slow things down a little?

Dorsal Vagal

- I see how down you've been. Have you ever tried sighing purposefully to relieve stress? It's actually a vagus nerve exercise to help people when they feel shut down.
- I know you want to sleep again. Can you sit on this harder chair so you don't nod off?
- How about we do an activity so you can stay a little more engaged? I'll throw this ball to you after I share and then you throw it back when you're finished talking and want a response.

Challenge Activities

SNS

- You're going so fast, I think you could burn out. How about we slow down, at least here. Lean on the wall, have some tea, or take a load off for a while. Do you feel any better just taking a pause?
- You have a lot of adrenaline keeping you awake. How would it be to put your hand over your beating chest and give it a little pressure. Soften your knees or feel your lower body. With some containment and grounding, does anything change with some time?
- Sounds like you've been going, going, going. Do you feel that sense of movement even though you're just sitting here? Is there a slower movement or stretch that might help you move that charge in a different way?
- Can you tense and release your body a few times and see if you relax a little more?

Dorsal Vagal

- Procrastination is the worst. When you feel that way next time, let's take a walk.
- Feeling stuck like that is challenging. Try this tapping with me. Then let's orient through our five senses. Do you feel any more alert or different after doing this activity?
- Next time you feel stuck, try moving your joints. Get out of immobility by challenging it.

- You're feeling so tired a lot of the time. How about we stroll around and talk a few minutes? We can walk in the office or a little outside and just connect with the environment around us. Sometimes movement and presence can be helpful when you're feeling so down.

> **Using the Polyvagal Promotions Protocol with Patients' Family Members**
>
> Everyone responds to feeling respected and to cues of belonging. Welcoming family members as your patients' advocates and appreciating their presence and intentions is a good way to establish the tone. Then consider the Polyvagal Promotions Protocol:
> 1. What is your polyvagal state and is there anything you need to do for yourself to connect to a ventral vagal state?
> 2. Interpret the family member's polyvagal state? You can hear this in their delivery of the interaction. For example, if they are upset, they are running in a high SNS tone. Sometimes it's embedded in the description, however. The person sounds very calm, but they are talking about something stressful and overwhelming. You might guess there is SNS tone that they might not be expressing to you.
> 3. In a ventral vagal state people want to feel listened to and taken seriously. So, the STAY protocol is usually most helpful at first. In psychology we call these "reflective comments." They are a part of practicing mirroring. You mirror, or reflect, the person's polyvagal state.
> 4. Try to come up with a solution to the problem. Start with a CHANGE comment, such as "This sounds upsetting, let me try to do something that will help" or "I hear that you've been very frustrated and care about your loved one; let me see what steps we can take to address some of the issues."
> 5. A CHALLENGE comment may be needed at some time: "I want to hear you, but I am wondering if you can slow down a little so I can better understand how to help you."
> 6. If the person enters a more ventral vagal state at any time, see if you can make a STAY-oriented comment to support the continuation of that polyvagal state, such as "I hear you saying it's not better yet but you're grateful to have the service here for your family member/significant other. We are glad you're reaching out so we can hear how to better serve your loved one."
> 7. Sometimes you need to leave the interaction even if you haven't satisfied the family member's need or request. Try to use your ventral vagal interaction as a part of the solution, such as "We heard you and I'll let my supervisor know, or we at the office know, how important billing disputes can be. We've added your comments to our ongoing records. We are not able to change the bill amount at this time; however, reaching out to us to let us know how that impacts you is important. If we can make the adjustment you requested, we will let you know. You can reach out to our finance department too."

Acute Risk and Crisis: Suicidal, Homicidal, Agitated, and Threatening Behaviors

When there is acute risk and crisis, it is important to remember that your survival physiology will be activated. If your patient is suicidal, homicidal, agitated, or threatening, your body is designed to respond in a mobilized way. It's essential to allow the mobilization to act, respond, and protect while also maintaining some ventral vagal capacity. In a ventral vagal state, you will have the capacity to be empathetic.

Of course, if there is imminent risk that the person may harm themselves or others, physical safety is paramount and must be taken care of first. This may involve your facility's policies and procedures on physical or chemical restraint, as well as calling emergency services (security, police, etc.). If at any time you feel unsafe, it is critical to remove yourself from the situation and call for help when able to do so. Often facilities will have alarm systems that can be triggered to call for help.

Stay Comments

Tone of voice: Avoid sounding too agitated or too soft; keep it neutral and steady.

Body position: Maintain flexible muscle tone, ready to respond but not bracing. If there are physical signs of agitation, try to relax your body but also stay ready to respond as needed. Being too relaxed can be a mismatched state of response.

Eye contact: Sometimes direct eye contact is threatening; other times, it is important for connection and recognition. Direct eye contact can offer respect and care in some situations and cultures, whereas for others it may be experienced as uncomfortable. You can also look toward someone but use your peripheral vision to see them.

In these situations, STAY then moving into CHANGE comments/actions often works. We want to meet the polyvagal state of the other person in a safe and friendly way. This prevents the person from getting angry that they are being ignored or not taken seriously and avoids triggering an instinctive aggression response. For example, "Hey man, I hear we have some things we've got to help you deal with." You might be louder and have more positive emotion with strength behind it. Going in softly, such as saying "How can I help you sir?," is not matched to meet the patient's SNS charge.

Key Takeaways

- The integration of the PVT into contemporary healthcare represents both a formidable challenge and a promising opportunity. This endeavor is marked by a profound schism between cognitive and somatic psychology. Cognitive psychology traditionally emphasizes internal cognitive processes, often sidelining the role of the body in human behavior and mental health. In contrast, somatic psychology recognizes the intricate connection between the body and mind. The PVT, informing somatic psychology, addresses the neurophysiological impacts of stress and trauma. While cognitive interventions may fall short, somatic approaches such as SE offer promise in healing trauma's effects on the body. To truly integrate the PVT into healthcare, a paradigm shift is required, bridging the cognitive–somatic gap and acknowledging the body–mind connection's pivotal role in mental health and well-being.
- Implementing polyvagal-informed interventions for patients is a multifaceted process involving several steps: education, self-regulation, interoceptive awareness, individualized and group interventions, autonomic mapping, and creating cues of safety. These steps aim to empower patients and healthcare professionals to understand and regulate their ANS states, fostering emotional well-being.
- Sound therapy can activate the social engagement system (ventral vagal state). Activities such as the SSP have demonstrated positive results when used to assess and improve emotional regulation.
- Creating cues of safety involves nonverbal communication, architectural design, and environmental elements to promote a sense of safety.

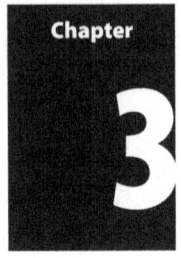

Chapter 3

Polyvagal-Informed HRM Policies and Procedures

Operating a healthcare organization, whether it be a small practice or a large hospital, requires policies and procedures that comply with regulations. In turning to human resources, we wondered how the PVT might inform this administrative aspect. This chapter narrows the focus in the healthcare arena to human resource management (HRM) activities, mostly focusing on recruitment and selection. We begin with a discussion of the root causes of bias and discrimination during the talent acquisition process. We then look at a broad range of implicit and explicit biases in the workplace. The chapter concludes with several practical recommendations for eliminating potential sources of bias and discrimination to assemble and cultivate a healthcare team that reflects diversity and inclusivity.

Objectives
- To understand the impact of stress and trauma on employee recruitment and selection activities.
- To clarify the common sources of implicit and explicit bias during the talent acquisition process.
- To identify practical polyvagal-informed strategies for eliminating bias and discrimination in HRM.

> **Scenario: Bias and Discrimination When Recruiting New Talent**
>
> Dr. Priya Cole is a seasoned healthcare professional with an impressive leadership track record, overseeing the clinic's operations and its team of dedicated medical practitioners. In her role as chief medical officer at Safe Haven, she is acutely aware of the demanding nature of the healthcare industry. The pressures, expectations, and emotional challenges healthcare professionals face are well known, making stress and trauma common occurrences in the field.
>
> Dr. Cole recognizes the vital role employee recruitment and selection activities play in maintaining a resilient and high-performing healthcare team. In her pursuit of equitable and inclusive recruitment, Dr. Cole is committed to identifying the sources of implicit and explicit bias that may influence the talent acquisition process. She aims to uncover how biases rooted in stress and trauma can inadvertently shape hiring decisions. She is determined to promote a discrimination-free recruitment process.
>
> Dr. Cole recognizes the value of polyvagal-informed strategies to create an inclusive and supportive work environment. She aspires to identify and implement practical approaches that can effectively eliminate bias and discrimination in HRM. By leveraging her position as chief medical officer, she intends to champion these strategies to create a healthcare team that thrives on diversity and inclusivity.

The Impact of Bias and Discrimination on Recruitment and Selection

The recruitment and selection process is a crucial gateway for securing top-tier doctors, nurses, therapists, specialists, and admin workers. It is the collective responsibility of healthcare leaders and the HR professionals in the industry to acknowledge that biases exist within the organization and to pave the way for equitable and inclusive recruitment.

For many years, bias has been a pervasive challenge in recruitment and possesses the power to undermine even the most robust HR management strategies. Although bias frequently occurs in hidden ways, it can worsen discrimination in the workplace, giving rise to cases where candidates are unjustly treated based on race, gender, religion, ethnicity, or national origin.

The use of heuristics (mental shortcuts) in social decision-making can be linked to the PVT's concept of neuroception (see Chapter 1: "Neuroception and Interoception"), whereby our nervous system rapidly evaluates cues in the environment, such as facial expressions, vocal tone, and body language. Heuristics allow for quick categorization of individuals based on these observable traits, which can lead to automatic judgments of others (Reihl et al. 2015). The repercussions of bias and discrimination often culminate in costly legal disputes with stakeholders, so it is important for healthcare leaders to take precautionary measures to prevent such occurrences.

Furthermore, research reveals that bias and discrimination are strongly related to a person's intuitive assessment of others. For example, researcher Miles and Sadler-Smith (2014) contend that many recruiters and managers rely heavily on their intuition and personal discretion when evaluating potential candidates. This propensity to trust one's instincts often hinges on what psychologists refer to as System 1 thinking. System 1 thinking is characterized by subjectivity, affectivity, intuition, and reflexive mechanisms, whereas System 2 thinking encompasses rational, analytical, and reflective dimensions, which are crucial for effective problem-solving.

The challenge arises when stress and trauma exert a significant influence on the decision-making process by pushing it toward quicker and habit-based System 1 thinking. Approximately 40% of senior managers in the United States rely on intuition to make personnel-related decisions, including hiring and interviewing (Miles and Sadler-Smith 2014). While intuition may occasionally yield favorable outcomes, it reduces the credibility of recruitment and selection activities, thereby worsening bias and discrimination.

In addition, it is crucial to mention that some candidates are inherently vulnerable to bias and discrimination. Recruiters are tasked to evaluate job applicants who are often strangers to them by relying on concise résumés and job applications to make long-term HRM decisions. As society increasingly focuses on gender equality and equal opportunities, unaddressed biases continue to undermine well-meaning initiatives. The presence of these biases can exacerbate disparities, making it more challenging for marginalized groups to access the same opportunities and positions as their counterparts. This problem can hinder societal progress and create obstacles for healthcare facilities that are striving to establish diverse and inclusive workforces. Thus, leaders and HR managers must proactively implement measures to address and mitigate the detrimental influence of bias and discrimination in recruitment and selection.

Sources of Bias and Discrimination

Bias and discrimination can manifest in many forms due to the growing complexity of social dynamics, staff attitudes, and HRM practices. For a true grasp of the severity of HRM bias, it is imperative to distinguish between implicit and explicit biases so that they can be addressed accordingly.

Implicit bias operates on a subconscious level and is usually driven by automatic processes that can elude an individual's awareness (Daumeyer et al. 2019). These subconscious associations sometimes lie beyond our control. Often stemming from the interviewer's stress-related and trauma-informed experiences, these biases can influence decision-making processes and destroy fair recruitment and selection procedures.

In contrast, *explicit bias* tends to occur through conscious mechanisms, whereby individuals are aware of their prejudices and can rationalize them. Often more apparent than implicit bias, explicit bias describes the attitudes, beliefs, and stereotypes that many people have for a specific group of individuals. This type of discrimination is often associated with personal prejudice, toxic organizational culture, stereotypes, and low diversity.

The detrimental impact of both types of bias on employee recruitment and selection outcomes is a major cause for concern. The distinction between implicit and explicit bias is clarified in Figure 3.1.

Table 3.1 sets forth common forms of bias and discrimination that commonly manifest in the HRM landscape. Recognizing these diverse forms of bias and discrimination is crucial for addressing and mitigating their impact on workers and society and for promoting fairness, equity, and inclusivity.

IMPLICIT BIAS

Unconscious attitudes or stereotypes that affect our understanding, actions, and decisions without our awareness. These biases operate automatically and unintentionally, influencing our behavior despite our conscious beliefs.

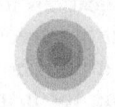

EXPLICIT BIAS

Conscious attitudes and beliefs that affect our understanding, actions, and decisions. These biases are deliberately formed and acknowledged, often expressed openly through words and actions.

VISIBLE

Figure 3.1 Defining implicit and explicit bias. As is shown, implicit bias is unconscious but influences behavior, and may escape conscious detection. (Source: authors.)

Table 3.1 Biases and discrimination in HRM

Type of Bias	How It Occurs	Example
Selective attention	Focusing on specific aspects while disregarding others that don't meet expected criteria.	Dr. Cole may inadvertently overlook applicants who don't exhibit the specific traits she values, such as resiliency and decisiveness. She might dismiss their potential without considering other valuable qualities they possess.
In-group bias	Favoring applicants from specific groups due to perceived affinity, shared traits, skills, or beliefs.	Dr. Cole may prefer candidates who share certain characteristics of hers. For instance, if she shares certain personality traits with an applicant, she may perceive them as a better fit for the clinic, potentially overlooking other candidates.
Overconfidence bias	Excessive confidence in one's ability to identify suitable candidates, often relying on intuition.	Dr. Cole may believe that her intuition about applicants is infallible, leading her to overlook potential hires. For instance, she may feel overly confident in her judgment, believing she can immediately spot the perfect candidate based on her gut feeling.
Appraisal bias	Assigning lower scores to individuals from minority groups based on subjective criteria.	Dr. Cole may undervalue the performance of minority candidates, assuming that factors like motherhood affect their commitment to work. This could result in a discriminatory recruitment process where capable candidates are unfairly judged.
Attributional bias	Making false assumptions about an applicant's performance based on perceived attributes.	Dr. Cole may wrongly judge candidates, thinking that certain traits or behaviors correlate with job performance. For example, she might assume that a candidate's shyness in an interview equates to an inability to excel in a healthcare role.
First-impression bias	Forming assumptions based on initial interactions, thereby leading to hasty judgments.	Dr. Cole may eliminate capable candidates due to their nervousness or first impressions during interviews. For instance, if a candidate appears nervous during an interview, she may assume they lack confidence, even though they may be qualified.
Confirmation bias	Selectively accepting information that aligns with preconceived notions while ignoring conflicting data.	Dr. Cole may favor applicants who match her expectations and dismiss data that challenges her beliefs. For example, if she has a preconceived notion that a candidate with a certain educational background is ideal, she may only consider information that supports this view.

Table 3.1 (cont.)

Type of Bias	How It Occurs	Example
Affinity bias	Preferring candidates who resemble the recruiter's traits, leading to subjective judgments.	Dr. Cole may lean toward applicants who mirror her characteristics, believing they are the best fit. For instance, if a candidate shares her interests, she may unconsciously favor them over others, regardless of their qualifications.
Projection bias	Believing others share the same goals, leading to misjudgments about candidate motivations.	Dr. Cole may misjudge candidates who have diverse motivations, assuming they align perfectly with the clinic's vision. For example, if a candidate is motivated by financial incentives rather than a deep commitment to healthcare, she might underestimate their potential contribution.
Halo and horn effects	Halo effect: Assuming proficiency in one area implies competence in all. Horn effect: Condemning candidates based on isolated flaws.	Dr. Cole may wrongly assess candidates, assuming that exceptional performance in one area signifies excellence in all aspects or rejecting candidates based on minor flaws. For instance, if a candidate excels in a specific skill, she might assume they are perfect for every aspect of the job.
Expectation anchor	Narrowing the recruitment process based on specific characteristics, limiting the candidate pool.	Dr. Cole may emphasize certain traits she believes are essential, thus excluding candidates with different qualities. For example, if she strongly believes that all applicants should be highly social and decisive, she may inadvertently exclude introverted but highly skilled candidates.
Conformity bias	Making conclusions influenced by peers and colleagues, aligning with popular opinions.	Dr. Cole may unconsciously let her colleagues' views affect her decisions during assessment meetings or group interviews. For instance, if her team expresses a strong preference for candidates with a specific background, she may conform to this view.
Contrast effect	Assessing candidates by comparing them to previous applicants, thereby causing biased judgments.	Dr. Cole may unfairly assess current candidates based on past applicants' performance, ignoring the unique potential of each individual. If previous recruits had specific characteristics, she might expect all candidates to possess the same traits, even if they are not relevant to the current job.

Table 3.1 (cont.)

Type of Bias	How It Occurs	Example
Taste-based discrimination	Developing preferences for certain applicant characteristics, such as physique or race.	Dr. Cole may show bias by favoring candidates who match her personal preferences instead of using structured, unbiased methods. For instance, if she prefers candidates with a certain appearance, she may unintentionally favor those candidates.
Statistical discrimination	Using statistical criteria to justify false perceptions about recruitment.	Dr. Cole may believe that specific population groups (based on statistics) are unsuitable for certain roles. For example, if she held a belief that workers from a particular demographic tend to be less productive, she would overlook a candidate from that group.

Polyvagal-Informed HRM Practices for Mitigating Bias and Discrimination

As many human resource managers recognize, recruitment and selection are dynamic and complex processes in any organization. With the emergence of new and revolutionary concepts regarding HRM, it is even more difficult for today's managers to understand whether their hiring decisions are based on subjective or objective considerations. In 2008, research revealed that approximately three out of four hiring managers prioritized subjective hiring decisions because they believed that they could "read between the lines" of the candidates' responses (Rozario et al. 2019).

Although considerable research has been performed on the critical factors that influence recruitment and selection, the reality is that there is no one-size-fits-all strategy for recruiting the perfect worker. This becomes increasingly challenging when the hiring manager is easily susceptible to bias and discrimination. Considering the evolution of human resource strategies, today's managers must acknowledge the strengths and weaknesses of relying on subjective versus objective measures when searching for new workers to add to their staff.

The underlying focus of this research is subjective decision-making because it is a notable cause of bias in the hiring process. While research points to significant improvements in reducing prejudice in the workplace, one of the most critical concerns is that many managers are unaware if their hiring decisions are, in fact, prejudicial.

The term "cognitive bias" emerged in 1972, when scientists discovered an unusual tendency of individuals to make systematic errors in their decision-making that are contrary to their rational choices (Thomas and Reimann 2023). For example, some leaders are influenced by their own overconfidence, while others are largely driven by overoptimism. Another common type of cognitive bias is the "ostrich effect," where one tends to ignore negative information by "burying one's head in the sand" (Thomas and Reimann 2023). These kinds of errors often lead to suboptimal outcomes.

The broad spectrum of biases and discrimination reveals that there are many situations where a human resources manager can unknowingly succumb to unfair hiring practices. Therefore, it is essential to increase human resources decision-makers' understanding of the large variety of cognitive biases and give them tools to reduce the potential pitfalls associated with biased hiring decisions.

Incidentally, each of these steps can also be applied to existing staff, with some modification.

1. Match the Candidates' Baseline State

The first polyvagal-informed strategy for eliminating bias and discrimination involves understanding and matching the candidates' autonomic state. According to Dana's findings in *Polyvagal Practices: Anchoring the Self in Safety* (2023), our autonomic state usually varies from protection to connection: protection describes the states of mobilization and immobilization (sympathetic and dorsal vagal, respectively); connection refers to the social engagement system (ventral vagal).

The ultimate sign of protection is being armored against others, whereas the ultimate sign of connection is being linked to another person. Being armored can present as an irritable or aggressive person who drives off others (sympathetic), or as withdrawal and avoidance (dorsal vagal). A person who is armored therefore may appear irritable, aggressive, or agitated, with rapid speech and movements (sympathetic), or quiet and withdrawn with minimal eye contact (dorsal vagal). This baseline is illustrated in Figure 3.2. In essence, most people live on a daily basis without knowing they are balancing between protection and connection. Nonetheless, there is a unique equilibrium at the center labeled "on the fence," where one is struggling between being safeguarded and being open to others. It is crucial to have an understanding of these stages to have a solid awareness of the candidates' baseline state. As a person is constantly pulled between the socialization, mobilization, and immobilization states, it becomes easier to create a more accurate autonomic profile that reflects their characteristics.

Based on this recommendation, managers need to match the candidates' emotional state to drive them to perform on the interview to their full potential. A candidates' categorization into the socialization, mobilization, or immobilization state is of the utmost

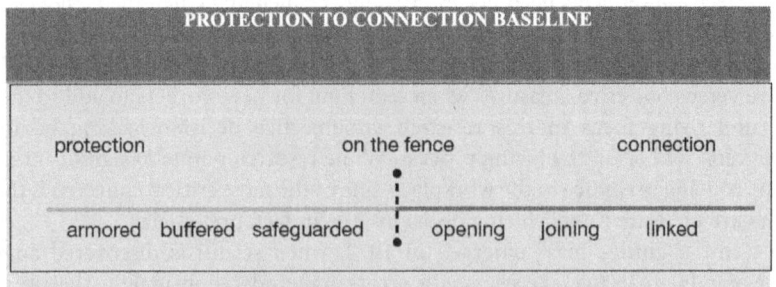

Figure 3.2 Autonomic baseline for protection and connection. Our willingness and comfort in connecting with others varies across a spectrum, based on our neuroception of whether there is a real or perceived threat. (Source: Dana 2023.)

priority because it can allow the manager to determine the most appropriate response for avoiding causing increased stress by an autonomic state mismatch.

- Candidates in the socialization state are often characterized by strong inclinations toward social engagement. Accordingly, most of these individuals excel in socialization and communication because their actions and decisions are positively influenced by their sympathetic state. These candidates will typically have good eye contact, appear relatively relaxed, and are friendly and not overly or avoidantly talkative. They display a natural curiosity and typically will freely provide information and ask questions.
- Candidates in the mobilization state tend to experience repetitive shifts across the polyvagal ladder. Accordingly, most of these individuals have a high disposition to perform the flight-or-flight response. These individuals are often anxious, nervous, impatient, or easily distracted in their respective workplaces. They can present with rapid speech and/or visible tremors, and may even become irritable. They also may appear to be too friendly or even somewhat impulsive.
- Candidates in the immobilization state are at the extreme end of the polyvagal ladder. Most of these individuals have a low tolerance for highly stressful situations because they often shut down when exposed to stressful circumstances. As such, immobilized individuals usually demonstrate lower energy levels compared to those in socialization or mobilization states.

Based on the three autonomic states, job descriptions should ideally be developed to understand the states that candidates fall under. These states may depend on the worker's temperament or their work responsibilities. With this knowledge, it is possible to determine the optimal positions or responsibilities for different workers. While some workers prefer to work as leaders, others tend to enjoy serving as frontline or back-end workers. Given that managers are usually considered the backbone of any organization, these workers are suitable for roles involving high social engagement.

High social engagement allows the managers to maintain good decision-making without fear of suddenly being mobilized or immobilized. In comparison, frontline workers often deal with large numbers of customers, so they often shift across the mobilization states. A good example of such an employee is a salesperson, who may often be required to deal with rude and aggressive customers.

With regard to the final autonomic state, individual candidates in the immobilization state are more suited for back-end roles because these positions are often less demanding than leadership or frontline roles. As a result, interviewers should ensure that workers who easily shift to immobilization be considered for positions in slower-paced environments.

Case Study 3.1: Improving Recruitment

Given Dr. Cole's commitment to equitable and inclusive recruitment practices and her recognition of the impact of stress and trauma on healthcare professionals, she can implement polyvagal-informed strategies to eliminate bias and discrimination in the talent acquisition process at Safe Haven Medical Clinic.

By comprehensively assessing the baseline autonomic states of potential hires, it will be possible to determine whether the individuals feel protected (mobilized or immobilized) or connected (socially engaged). Afterward, Dr. Cole can tailor recruitment efforts to match the individual preferences and temperaments of candidates. For instance, candidates inclined toward social engagement may excel in leadership roles, while those experiencing mobilization states may thrive in frontline positions, such as dealing with patients directly. Similarly, individuals with a propensity for immobilization may find back-end roles at the clinic more suitable. This approach ensures that each healthcare professional is placed in a role that aligns with their baseline autonomic state, thereby fostering a work environment conducive to optimal performance.

Although a person's state can shift over time, having an interview process with several touch points and observations can give a fairly accurate idea of what each candidate's baseline autonomic state may be. Of course, if the individual is hired and ends up displaying a different baseline state, then the manager and organization can work with that individual to either modify the job description or offer to train the worker on the self-regulation skills discussed in Chapter 1 (in the hope it will help them have some choice around which state they want to be in during work hours).

2. Identify Potential Inequalities

We have discussed how implicit and explicit biases can impact recruitment and selection of candidates. The human tendency is to group individuals into categories, and no discussion of this would be complete without addressing issues around equality. Wolgast et al. (2017) highlight that the categorization of workers into groups often causes negative perceptions between the in-group and out-group collectives. This can promote favoritism toward in-group members or result in the exclusion of out-group individuals.

Nonetheless, a significant gap facing existing research on staff inequality involves the inherent focus on singular dimensions of inequality, whereas the interplay of factors such as positional and relational power dynamics has been largely neglected. Rosicgno (2019) claims that research on workplace inequalities has developed in an insightful direction, but the failure to consider the interplay of specific factors that amplify prejudice is a critical weakness in understanding the problem. To address this issue, today's HR managers need to understand that body-related characteristics, such as race, gender, and age, are some of the most common vulnerabilities within the domains of hiring and employment (Rosicgno 2019). Let's look at each.

- **Ageism:** The evolution of healthcare and technology has contributed to a substantial improvement in overall health and life expectancy. As a result, the proportion of older workers and older candidates seeking jobs has increased, resulting in a more diversified workforce. However, this increasing diversity has worsened age-related conflicts in the workplace. There are many age-based stereotypes, such as that older workers are less productive, less adaptable, or less motivated than younger workers (Bae and Choi 2023). Incidentally, younger workers are not immune to ageism; these employees may face injustices during promotions or delegation of responsibilities due to the perception they are less experienced or less loyal than older workers (Bae and Choi 2023). Ageism is a multifaceted problem that emerges due to the segregation of workers according to their ages. Hiring managers have a crucial responsibility to ensure that neither population is subject to age-related discrimination.
- **Racial prejudice:** Unfortunately, many workers from diverse racial origins or minority ethnic communities are often segregated as outliers in their respective workplaces. This problem is particularly common among immigrants and members of Indigenous racial groups. Moreover, racial prejudice can also occur in more subtle forms. For instance,

Berry and Bell (2012) explain that it is common for some recruiters to place too much emphasis on the perceived "blackness" or the "whiteness" of the applicant's name. Similar claims were highlighted by Lancee (2021), who revealed that applicants with foreign-sounding names often need to send 5% more applications compared to equally qualified applicants from the majority racial group. Although significant efforts have been undertaken to eliminate racial prejudice, tackling implicit bias in the human resource sector is still a daunting (but not impossible) task.

- **Gender-based discrimination**: This tends to occur due to a person's gender or orientation. Traditionally, the workplace was considered inhospitable to women because they often faced numerous types of inequalities due to their sex. As a result, there was a scarcity of women in leadership roles, and this also increased the amount of time women required in order to advance in their respective careers (Stamarski and Hing 2015). On top of that, many women were stigmatized or experienced stress due to discrimination. Historically, this problem has contributed to significant social and economic gaps between men and women in the workplace. The most effective strategy for tackling institutional sexism is to reform the structures and processes that promote gender-based discrimination. This approach includes altering the leadership, organizational climate, vision, or HR policies to make the workplace more conducive to both men and women. Admittedly, the healthcare industry has made significant strides in being at the forefront of gender equality. Nonetheless, recruiters interviewing candidates should ensure they check for any explicit or implicit biases they may hold around gender.

While these are the three most common biases, candidates can be unfairly judged (and workers can be segregated) based on their sexual orientation, marital status, nationality, religion, or disability. Understanding the interplay of these factors can mitigate prejudice during the hiring process and in the workplace.

As a side note, recent studies reveal that workplace injustice can negatively impact disadvantaged populations (Okechukwu et al. 2014). Some workers may experience PTSD due to bullying, while others may demonstrate unstable emotional and psychological responses to real or perceived threats or criticism. Furthermore, not reporting experiences of discrimination can worsen the toll on the victim's health. Okechukwu et al. (2014) discovered this phenomenon among African American female workers who did not report instances of unfair treatment; they were four times more likely to develop high blood pressure than those who did report the injustices. Therefore, identifying vulnerable workers and eliminating causes of bias-based stress is essential to ensure positive mental, physical, and emotional outcomes for all employees.

Case Study 3.2: Improving Recruitment

Dr. Cole is strategically positioned to implement polyvagal-informed strategies for equitable and inclusive recruitment. She recognizes that healthcare professionals often face significant stress and trauma due to the demanding nature of their roles. By considering the interplay of factors that amplify prejudice, such as power dynamics and the diverse vulnerabilities of staff members, Dr. Cole adopts a holistic approach to recruitment.

This involves recognizing that age, race, gender, sexual orientation, marital status, nationality, religion, and disability should *not* influence hiring decisions. Dr. Cole aims to create a discrimination-free recruitment process, ensuring that candidates are evaluated based on their skills, qualifications, and potential contributions to the team.

3. Restructure the Hiring Process

An effective recommendation for mitigating bias and discrimination during the talent acquisition process is to introduce highly structured human resource practices. These practices can ensure that the hiring managers receive adequate information concerning the applicants instead of relying on subjective considerations.

In situations where the hiring manager has inadequate objective information concerning the applicants, the likelihood that they will rely on stereotypes or other biased decision-making mechanisms increases significantly (Wolgast et al. 2017). Therefore, it is essential to acquire adequate information to reduce the potential for bias and discrimination. There are various ways to increase the systematicity of the selection process (Wolgast et al. 2017). An example is comprehensive job analysis, which plays an important role in enhancing the integrity of talent acquisition procedures, such as examining, documenting, and making appropriate inferences about the job's requirements or the workers' attributes (Wolgast et al. 2017). These highly structured human resource practices are integral for creating a fair talent acquisition process that does not discriminate against candidates based on their individual characteristics. Although this recommendation does not fall under polyvagal-informed practices, it is a practical solution for eliminating critical weaknesses in recruitment and selection. By taking out some of the guesswork, the recruiter is better able to maintain a regulated state, which reduces the risk of making decisions based on implicit bias.

To reduce subjective decision-making, recruiters are recommended to combine tried-and-tested recruitment strategies with emerging approaches. When recruitment decisions are implicitly driven, there is a high likelihood that their rational control over selections will decline (Kroll et al. 2021). Classical recruitment strategies are the "gold standard" in recruitment because they are supported by considerable evidence. For instance, the use of CVs to screen applicants has been a reliable approach for assessing applicants for many decades. In comparison, modern recruitment strategies are highly dependent on human resource technologies, such as social network sites, external recruitment agencies, and active sourcing (Kroll et al. 2021). These sources provide as much information as the traditional approaches and they offer the recruiters more options, such as providing personality assessment options for applications. This explains why these recruitment approaches have gained significant traction. However, the underlying challenge facing today's approaches revolves around their reliance on automated decisions. By combining classic and emerging recruitment approaches, hiring managers can reduce their likelihood of making biased hiring decisions.

> **Case Study 3.3: Tackling Bias and Discrimination in Hiring**
>
> In addressing the challenge of bias and discrimination during the hiring process at Safe Haven Medical Clinic, Dr. Cole embraces a multifaceted approach that integrates highly structured human resource practices with classic and emerging recruitment strategies. The introduction of highly structured human resource practices becomes a cornerstone of her strategy. By ensuring that hiring managers receive comprehensive and objective information about applicants, this approach minimizes the likelihood of subjective considerations and reliance on stereotypes.

To further reduce susceptibility to subjective bias, Dr. Cole incorporates a combination of tried-and-tested recruitment strategies with emerging approaches. Combining classic and emerging recruitment approaches allows Dr. Cole to strike a balance that reduces the potential for biased hiring decisions. By having a clear framework to minimize bias and maintain a regulated state of social engagement, Dr. Cole recognizes its practical significance in eliminating critical weaknesses in the clinic's talent acquisition practices.

4. Create Accurate Job Descriptions Based on Polyvagal States

To eliminate bias and discrimination, healthcare organizations need to abandon subjective processes and focus on practices that prioritize the applicants' competency, character, and work experience. An article published in the *Harvard Business Review* explains that most traditional job descriptions are unable to keep up with the rate of change in modern job roles (Nieto-Rodriguez 2023).

There are many situations where healthcare organizations begin the recruitment process without fully understanding the job's roles and requirements. For example, a company may recruit an employee to perform a specific set of tasks, but four months later a different set of tasks becomes the priority. Even if the workers possess the right skills for the new tasks, they may lack the ability to adapt to the change. Changes in job roles can cause significant stress among employees and reduce their performance levels. Some job descriptions are created to search for prospective applicants, while others are designed to serve as a benchmark for assessing employee performance or planning employee development (Nieto-Rodriguez 2023). For organizations to drive their workers to perform to their full potential, they need to clarify the descriptions of vacant positions.

The PVT can also be incorporated into the decision-making process to create effective job descriptions. When creating a job description, the designer needs to deliberate whether it should be outcome-focused, skill-focused, or team-based. We can anticipate that an individual's autonomic state at a given moment will impact their fit with one of these subcategories, as discussed next.

- Outcome-focused job descriptions require the company to specify the expected outcomes of the position. For instance, Google follows the belief that "When employees know what is expected of them and how they will be measured, they are more likely to be motivated and engaged in their work" (Nieto-Rodriguez 2023). Outcome-oriented job descriptions are more convenient for workers in demanding positions with strict requirements. This is particularly helpful in roles such as performing procedures in a surgical area or intensive care units with a high degree of algorithms.
- Skill-focused job descriptions usually outline the skills and capabilities that the employee should bring to the table. Accordingly, these descriptions shift the focus from the employees' responsibilities to their individual talents and proficiencies. Skill-focused descriptions are more favorable for versatile workers who have broad skill sets. In the healthcare setting, this would include those who problem-solve diagnosis and treatment, and who can synthesize a wide range of information into diagnostic formulations.
- Team-based job descriptions indicate the responsibilities of the members of the team. For example, Spotify uses this model, whereby its employees work as cross-functional

teams called "squads" (Nieto-Rodriguez 2023). Team-based descriptions are more appropriate for workers who need to remain in the social engagement state. This would include customer service and front desk employees, as well as those involved in quality and utilization management.

Taking these insights into consideration, accurate job descriptions reflect a healthcare facility's fair and unbiased talent acquisition processes. By matching autonomic state with appropriate job roles, we can expect more satisfied and productive staff who enjoy their positions.

> **Case Study 3.4: Optimizing Job Descriptions**
>
> Dr. Cole leverages her role as chief medical officer to create a more equitable recruitment process that emphasizes the importance of accurate job descriptions. While designed to attract prospective applicants, job descriptions can also be used as benchmarks for assessing performance and to plan employee development. In this way, accurate and purposeful job descriptions become the cornerstone of driving employees to perform to their full potential.
>
> By aligning job descriptions with the polyvagal state and recognizing the need for accuracy and clarity in defining roles, Dr. Cole positions Safe Haven Medical Clinic to adopt fair and unbiased talent acquisition processes. This proactive approach not only addresses bias and discrimination but also contributes to an inclusive workplace environment that supports employee well-being and maximizes performance.

5. Cultivate an Organizational Culture with Less Stress and Trauma

Healthcare leadership has an ethical responsibility to create healthy and trauma-free environments for their employees in order to provide cues of safety that help workers regulate their ANS. This begins with the development of a supportive organizational culture.

To provide some background, "organizational culture" describes the way employees perform assigned tasks and interact with others in the workplace (Kim and Jung 2022). This culture can serve as a symbol for or reflect the values shared by most workers within the organization. As a result, a solid organizational culture can allow for open communication and shared decision-making. In current times, positive organizational culture has been commonly associated with increased inclusion and diversity, which again begins with the hiring process. When workers feel valued for their unique qualities and contributions, they can develop a sense of belonging that reduces their likelihood of judging others based on race, age, and gender biases.

Research reveals that the main types of organizational cultures are hierarchy, clan, adhocracy, and market cultures (Crandall and Crandall 2008). Foremost, the hierarchy culture highlights the importance of a rigid structure and levels of authority among the workers. We tend to see this in many healthcare settings, such as hospitals and outpatient clinics, that perform numerous procedures. Clan culture encourages workers to view each other as a close-knit family with a strong common interest. This tends to be more dominant in small group and private practice settings, as well as behavioral health organizations. Adhocracy is more flexible and is less focused on bureaucracy and innovation. Given the high degree of regulation in healthcare, this would be less common, but might be seen in peer-run support services that provide

Types of **Organizational Culture**

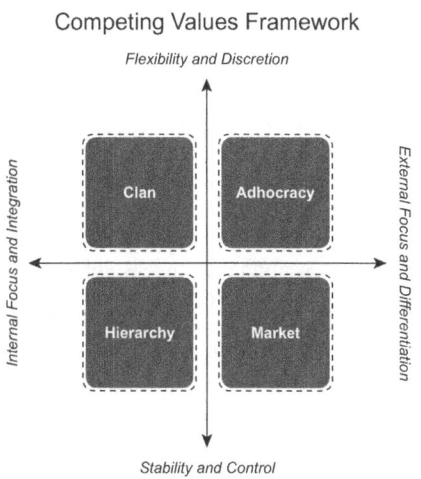 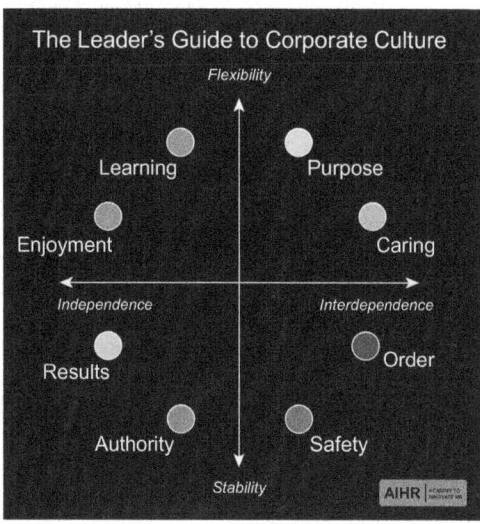

Figure 3.3 Types of organizational culture. (Source: Gardner 2023.)

educational groups and general support for clients. The market culture is relatively unique because it concentrates on adaptation, maximizing profits, and staying ahead of the competition. This would be most prevalent in cosmetic service organizations such as medi-spa and plastic surgery clinics. The main features of these organizational cultures are illustrated in Figure 3.3.

Unfortunately, it can be quite challenging to change existing workers' beliefs and values to create a culture that is conducive to diversity, inclusion, feelings of safety, adaptation, and worker satisfaction. In fact, Kim and Jung (2022) recognize that altering the culture is one of an organization's most challenging tasks because workers may be too accustomed to the previous culture to adapt to new requirements. What's more, they may feel threatened by new hires and interoffice restructuring that doesn't align with their preconceptions of what the workplace should be.

In alignment with the PVT, Parent and Lovelace (2018) outline four potential responses to change and trauma: succumb, survive, be resilient, or thrive. The drive to succumb is the lowest level of change and corresponds with the immobilization state (dorsal vagal), whereas the survive and be resilient responses match the mobilization state (sympathetic). Finally, the thrive response corresponds with the social engagement state (ventral vagal). With this in mind, healthcare leadership can alter how the staff responds and behaves by encouraging them to adapt and thrive in the face of perceived threats and danger. The organization needs to implement strategic and gradual efforts to effect a positive cultural shift in the workers' values. This begins with polyvagal-informed strategies that can help strengthen the staff's mental and emotional resilience.

> **Case Study 3.5: Creating a Supportive Work Culture**
>
> The recommendation to cultivate a workplace culture with less drama, stress, and trauma resonates with the ethical responsibility of creating an environment that supports the well-being of healthcare professionals. To achieve this alignment, Safe Haven Medical Clinic must implement initiatives that encourage employees to adapt and thrive in the face of threats and challenges.
>
> For instance, Dr. Cole can emphasize the importance of creating a good work–life balance by encouraging the staff to balance their time at work and their time off effectively. This balance can play a vital role in improving their well-being and overall satisfaction at work. She can also create a wellness program that is explicitly designed to alter the organization's culture and fulfill the employees' physical and mental needs.
>
> Dr. Cole acknowledges that a robust organizational culture serves to reflect shared values among the staff. Most importantly, a positive organizational culture is linked to increased inclusion and diversity, fostering an environment wherein everyone feels valued for their unique qualities and contributions. This, in turn, reduces the likelihood of biased judgments based on race, age, or gender. By aligning the corporate culture with the PVT, Safe Haven Medical Clinic will strengthen staff awareness of social engagement and safety.

Key Takeaways

- The employee recruitment and selection process are largely based on the recruiter's ability to make accurate decisions based on subjective and objective measures. However, bias and discrimination can undermine a facility's ability to recruit the best employees. Proactive measures need to be undertaken to prevent an organization from recruiting workers who may fail to deliver optimally or that may result in costly legal disputes. Given the large number of recruiters who rely on their intuition and the large number of vulnerable employees, organizations need to adopt proactive measures for mitigating biases and discrimination while fostering inclusive environments.
- Bias and discrimination occur in both subtle and overt ways. Implicit bias occurs when a person makes prejudicial decisions without conscious awareness. In such scenarios, they are driven by automatic mental processes. Explicit bias occurs through conscious means, whereby the individual has full awareness of their prejudice. Understanding how to tackle these biases can drastically improve the success of an organization's HRM activities.
- The application of PVT concepts can eliminate critical weaknesses in modern HRM practices. Healthcare professionals can use polyvagal-informed strategies to eliminate implicit and explicit prejudices and improve HRM decisions. First, understanding the employees' autonomic state can provide recruiters with a benchmark for determining whether applicants are inclined to the socialization, mobilization, or immobilization states and thus make optimal decisions around matching candidates with suitable job descriptions. Second, identifying candidates and employees who may be marginalized can eliminate instances of bias in the selection process and in the workplace. Third, restructuring the talent acquisition process and reformulating job descriptions can promote objective hiring decisions. And fourth, transforming the corporate culture can create a stress-free environment that fosters adaptability, diversity, inclusion, and well-being.

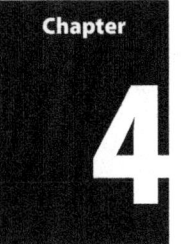

Chapter 4: Leadership and Management in Healthcare

From the ER to the switchboard, healthcare settings are often highly stressful, to varying degrees. Continuous stress can affect both the medical and support staff, leading to health complaints, reduced workflow, and poor interpersonal relationships. This chapter delves into strategies for leading and managing workers in these mentally, emotionally, and physically demanding environments. It is management's job to ensure that workers can perform at their best when faced with work-related challenges and changing circumstances. While polyvagal-informed strategies improve outcomes in the workplace, leaders and managers are integral factors in employee productivity and well-being. This chapter presents a comprehensive evaluation of common leadership styles that may be employed by healthcare organizations and investigates team-based leadership strategies.

Objectives
- To examine the cause of work-related stressors and their effects on healthcare workers.
- To identify the most effective leadership styles for healthcare professionals in high-stress roles.
- To understand how to build strong, resilient, and efficient teams.
- To analyze innovative methods to optimize employee outcomes in individual and team settings.

> **Scenario: Navigating the Leadership Storm at Safe Haven**
>
> Safe Haven Medical Clinic has always had a reputation for delivering high-quality care to patients. As the chief medical officer, Dr. Cole has a responsibility to provide leadership and oversight for all clinical matters, which she has successfully done for several years.
>
> However, now that the clinic is experiencing unprecedented surges in incoming patients, a significant amount of pressure has been placed on the staff. Many workers have noticed a drastic surge in their tasks and responsibilities, leading them to work longer hours and take shorter breaks. What's more, continuously dealing with patients who are suffering to some degree has been taking an emotional toll on them. Many of the staff members have reported high stress levels and a few have hinted that they might resign.
>
> These emerging issues encouraged Dr. Cole to switch leadership styles, knowing that the right leadership style can strengthen the relationship between staff and management. This requires her to understand the variety of leadership approaches and their relevance to the clinic's needs.
>
> Among these approaches are transactional, transformational, situational, and servant leadership styles. Dr. Cole's current leadership style is transactional, which prioritizes the clinic's chain of command and praises/reprimands employees based on their performance. Now, however, she will consider how other leadership styles might improve the situation.

She also plans to re-evaluate the characteristics of the work teams and the team leaders to ensure they are still a good fit in light of the rising stress levels. Once those steps are complete, Dr. Jennings will incorporate more polyvagal-informed strategies into the workplace.

Stress and Trauma in the Healthcare Setting

Exposure to stress and trauma is an unavoidable part of working in the healthcare sector. This exposure begins as early as school, where students first lay eyes on cadavers or gruesome injuries, and progresses as they become seasoned professionals. Hence, the nature of the healthcare environment allows healthcare professionals to experience all kinds of traumatic events, which can occur on a day-to-day basis or during rare events, such as during disasters (Morganstein et al. 2017). For many healthcare workers, this type of learning allows them to become more resilient to trauma as they progress.

Considerable literature has been published concerning the scope of the problem, and the main finding is that healthcare workers respond differently to work-associated stress and trauma. Research by Rink et al. (2023) notes that at least 70% of healthcare workers experience high stress and burnout, which can easily hinder patient care. Stress levels have increased in recent years due to disasters such as the COVID-19 pandemic. In this published research, the authors identified that up to 70% of nurses and 30% of physicians reported high stress levels during the study period. Moreover, nurses recorded a 40.6% rate of emotional exhaustion in 2019; this surged to 49.2% in 2022 (Rink et al. 2023). The rise was largely attributable to the pandemic, and thus a wide variety of strategies have emerged that aim to promote the health and mental well-being of healthcare workers in order to help them be more resilient to stress and trauma.

In essence, many individuals exposed to stress and trauma emerge with limited or no adverse effects. These individuals resume their social and occupational roles due to their high resilience (Morganstein et al. 2017). However, some people experience a reduction in their sense of competence, their self-efficacy, and their belief that they can manage future stressors. Furthermore, a sizable minority demonstrate adverse psychological and behavioral responses in the form of distress reactions, psychiatric disorders, and health risk behaviors. Figure 4.1 highlights these responses to traumatic stress.

Research reveals that approximately 10–20% of individuals who are exposed to traumatic events develop PTSD; however, a large number also show mild symptoms, which can easily persist and escalate (Morganstein et al. 2017). Although PTSD is not the only trauma-related disorder, it is the most common. Healthcare workers may also experience generalized anxiety disorder, panic disorder, or increased substance abuse. In brief, there is a dose-related response to traumatic events, which increases the likelihood of developing traumatic stress. Given this problem, healthcare organizations need to make workers' health and well-being a top priority.

Distress reactions are cited as the most common outcome of consistent exposure to stress and trauma. For instance, many individuals feel anger and an increased sense of vulnerability after a traumatic event, while others become demoralized or lose faith (Morganstein et al. 2017). It is also common for these individuals to experience insomnia and irritability, and to become easily distracted. Some people display physical symptoms or psychological distress, resulting in somatic complaints such as headaches, dizziness, fatigue,

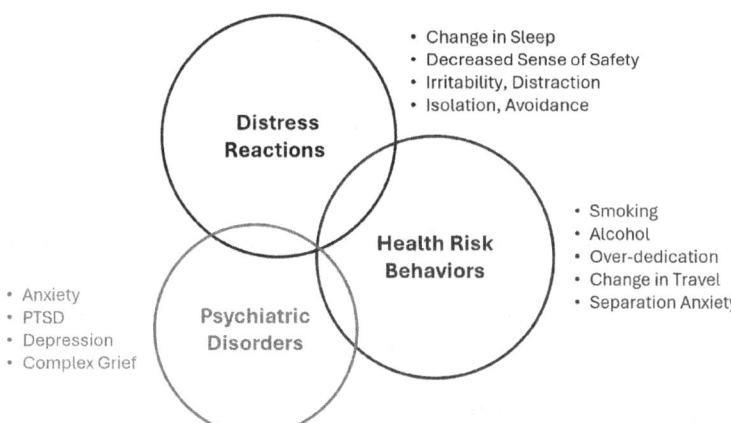

Figure 4.1 Physiological and behavioral responses to traumatic stress. The diagram shows how exposure to stressful events can impact behavior and mental health. (Source: Morganstein et al. 2017, 36.)

nausea, and general weakness. There are many cases where physical disorders cannot be easily identified because the distress reaction occurs irregularly. Other reactions include a decreased sense of safety, isolation, and avoidance. Awareness of these distress reactions is crucial to prevent the traumatic stress from escalating.

In comparison, psychiatric disorders can manifest following consistent exposure to trauma. These disorders include anxiety, PTSD, depression, and complex grief. Research reveals that there are some events that amplify traumatic stress, such as the duration and intensity of exposure to a traumatic event (Morganstein et al. 2017): prolonged exposure to a traumatic event can increase one's chances of developing traumatic stress. For example, natural disasters often generate lower levels of impairment compared to events such as mass violence. Similarly, high-impact traumatic events can worsen a healthcare worker's psychiatric response. In particular, events that result in significant uncertainty about the potential risks, such as infectious diseases and exposure to harmful radiation, tend to carry widespread and lasting psychological effects. Furthermore, continuous exposure to traumatic events increases the likelihood of developing a psychiatric disorder. For example, a vascular surgeon who amputates the limb of a single patient is less likely to develop traumatic stress than one who amputates seven limbs following a terrorist blast. Although the science of safety is still unclear, there are many psychiatric disorders associated with consistent exposure to stress and trauma.

Regarding health risk behaviors, the aftermath of a traumatic event often triggers various behaviors. For example, one prevalent response is an increase in a person's tendency to abuse substances such as alcohol, tobacco, caffeine, or medications (Morganstein et al. 2017). These actions are often undertaken as a form of self-medication to alleviate the symptoms of traumatic stress. While this may provide a sense of relief, it can contribute to long-term health effects. Moreover, it is common for some people to develop a diminished sense of safety, encouraging them to avoid other people or avoid travel away from their home. These responses result from an increased sense of vulnerability, which encourages a person to cope through isolation or avoidance. Furthermore, some individuals become more violent following exposure to trauma, which can make them prone to intimate partner violence or community violence. Significant research points to a strong correlation between traumatic stress and violence.

While healthcare workers may demonstrate different health risk behaviors from those mentioned here, any of these maladaptive behaviors can negatively affect performance and productivity at work.

Practical Leadership Styles for the Healthcare Environment

Leadership style is "a set of regular behaviors and activities that characterize the daily relationship between the manager and the person below him in the corporate hierarchy, the manager's conscious behavior toward employees who are dependent on him, and the manager's perception and actions of people management" (Arany and Popovics 2022, 92). From another perspective, leadership style can mean the leader's ability to exercise power, including the methods they use to influence their workers. It can also mean the leader's approach to ensure alignment between the workers and the organization's goals.

Practical leadership styles are vital for allowing healthcare facilities and organizations to navigate through the complex challenges that are inherent to the healthcare environment. According to Arany and Popovics (2022), the history of leadership can be compared to human evolution. Since the dawn of humankind, certain human beings have demonstrated unique attitudes, qualities, and behaviors that compel others to put them in power and follow them. While there is considerable diversity in the terms used for those in leadership throughout time, what has remained constant is the leadership role.

Our current understanding of leadership is supported by centuries of research. In the 1940s and 1950s, many scholars sought to identify the most important traits leaders should possess. Due to the broad spectrum of leadership styles and organizational needs, the findings were not conclusive.

Since the nineteenth century, the main questions have been as follows: Who is a leader? Are good leaders born or made? What makes a good leader? Should organizations prioritize leaders who have excellent professional skills, communication skills, management skills, or courage? How do aspects such as patience, empathy, and understanding impact leadership outcomes? Given these questions, it is clear that there is no one-size-fits-all approach to leadership that can satisfy all situations. Still, considering that today's leaders are often selected from the most qualified, experienced, or inspiring individuals, it remains important to understand the traits embraced by these individuals.

While there are no conclusive answers to these questions, leadership has continued to grow as a field of research. For instance, Hunt and Fedynich (2019) try to clarify the controversy by providing two perspectives: (1) Some researchers argue from the basis of whether good leaders are born with an innate ability to lead or whether these skills can be cultivated and nurtured. This viewpoint implies that individuals who exhibit leadership traits at an early age, such as charisma and decisiveness, are naturally predisposed to become leaders in later life. And (2), a small group of extremists contend that leadership is a fictional construct. These critics believe that leadership is a subjective and socially constructed concept without a tangible basis. As such, leadership should be perceived as a label assigned by a social or organizational entity.

For our purpose, leadership development in the healthcare sector is perceived as a continuum where a person begins by achieving several milestones that are synonymous

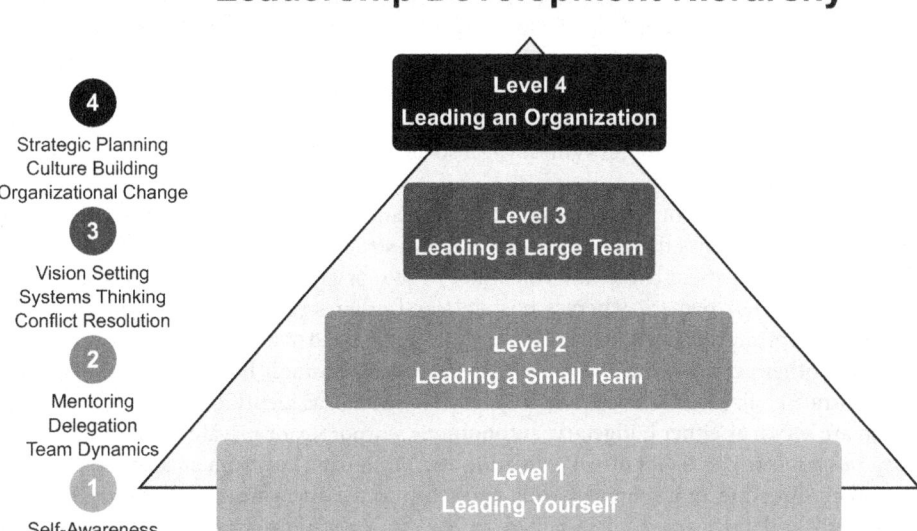

Figure 4.2 Basic hierarchy model for leadership development. (Source: authors.)

with good leadership. Foremost, one begins by developing a basic mastery of one's strengths, weaknesses, and foundational skills. This knowledge is essential for allowing a leader to comprehend how to incorporate themselves into teams and the broader organization. The next stage is to understand how to lead different types of teams. Fundamentally, small teams may consist of 3 to 10 members, whereas large teams may range from 10 to 50 individuals. In small teams, leaders require good management and leadership skills to identify how to optimize the team's overall performance. With this knowledge, one can transition into managing large teams and subteams. After developing basic competency in these areas, the leader can consider progressing to organizational leadership. Leading an organization requires one to know how to coordinate several teams simultaneously. This step of the hierarchy marks the mastery of the basic milestones of leadership development (see Figure 4.2).

Leading Workers in High-Stress Healthcare Environments

Many organizations recognize that leadership is a critical factor in their overall success or failure. As such, the traditional leadership style, where the leader serves as the boss and sole decision-maker, has gradually been eliminated in favor of more efficient leadership styles. Given that leaders are usually nominated to provide direction and build their teams, they need to understand how to create a conducive work environment for all workers. Arany and Popovics (2022, 21) claim that "a business can grow as high as its leader can grow." According to these researchers, it does not matter whether the organization is a small, medium, or large enterprise; in all cases, the qualities and traits of the leaders are vital for an enterprise's overall success. Thus, professional proficiency and a solid understanding of leadership are essential for enabling positive change in all organizations. Healthcare organizations need to employ good leaders to stimulate their workers and push them to their full potential. This helps the organization to showcase itself as a safe, compassionate place for individuals to receive excellent healthcare, and to attract highly skilled professionals who serve the community and increase healthy outcomes locally. By providing cues of safety, the healthcare leadership promotes ventral vagal socialization and helps to promote well-being and connection.

Before we address concepts around leadership and how the PVT can inform these, it is useful to briefly discuss the various organizational structures that healthcare facilities may deploy. Many outpatient clinics are run either as solo or group practices, with one or more managing partners/owners, whereas hospitals and other large entities are typically a for-profit or nonprofit corporation. This includes executive leadership and a board of directors, as well as other executives who oversee their respective business lines.

Khosravi et al. (2022) describe four types of hospitals, as identified by the World Bank, which are set up as either budgetary, autonomous, corporate, or private entities. Budgetary hospitals tends to run under direct regulation and input from government agencies, whereas the other three are more aligned with marketization. How a healthcare organization is structured and the personnel recruited to lead its operations have a direct impact on corporate community, culture, and leadership. Specifically, there are various ways in which an organization can develop cues of safety or danger and impact the ANS state of employees and patients. One could argue that government oversight might be seen as a cue for safety to some and for danger to others!

The key leadership styles emphasized in this section for helping workers navigate through high-stress environments are transactional, transformational, situational, and servant leadership. Each has its inherent strengths and weaknesses, so leaders need to understand which approach is more effective for their respective work settings. As we review these leadership styles, think about which autonomic state on the polyvagal ladder each might promote, in both workers and clients. This again leads to the concept of providing cues of safety and connection, as a means to shift away from any sympathetic mobilization or dorsal vagal immobilization states.

Transactional Leadership

The transactional leadership style is one of the oldest leadership styles in history. It is consistent with the use of rational decision-making faculties, so it can provide essential information about perceived danger and safety. Potter and Starcke (2022) explain that transactional leadership usually occurs when the leader exchanges something with economic, political, or psychological value with their followers. In healthcare, we can see examples of leaders who report on productivity and claims revenue generated by each staff member who can bill for their services, for example.

Transactional leadership requires the leader to act as an authoritarian and to create a highly structured chain of command for their workers. For that reason, leaders often expect their employees to comply with the organization's rules and regulations. Another unique trait of transactional leadership involves low personal identification between leaders and their staff, making leaders who use this style seem machine-like. This is more apparent in organizations that rely on procedures and algorithms, such as surgical centers or intensive care units. From a PVT perspective, a blend of ventral vagal and sympathetic states is seen as most common, providing some level of communication with an emphasis on independent mobilization (staff are expected to be able to function autonomously but follow the rules).

Transactional leadership can be further categorized into two classifications: active management by exception and passive management by exception (Aga 2016). Active management by exception is a form of management where the transactional leader prioritizes purely functional work interactions. In other words, aspects that are work-related are given precedence, whereas aspects that are not work-related are seen as excessive. Passive management by exception involves the leader actively supervising the workers and providing corrective action after a problem occurs. As a result, these leaders are often highly attentive to their workers during problems or adverse events. Although these approaches are somewhat different, they share a similarity in terms of low identification between the leader and the subordinates.

In addition, this style is highly dependent on the distribution of rewards and punishments to stimulate workers to perform to their fullest. The transactional approach is based on the idea that employees are primarily driven by extrinsic motivation. These remunerations usually come in the form of financial rewards, promotions, status, recognition, support, company perks such as a preferred schedule and flexible paid days off, or financial assistance for continuing education and licensure reimbursement. As such, the use of positive and negative reinforcement should serve the goal of stimulating workers to deliver their full potential at work. However, the inherent nature of the transactional leadership style can easily result in increased adverse reactions, such as severe stress and anxiety for workers. The low emphasis on intrinsic motivation is a key obstacle in this leadership style because it can create a workplace that does not support social engagement.

Lyons and Schneider (2009) compared the costs and benefits of the transformational and transactional leadership approaches on employees' stress outcomes. According to these scholars, leaders who advocate for supportive relationships between the workers often promote employee motivations and facilitate more positive emotional connections between them. This explains why the transformational leadership style tends to demonstrate better outcomes than the transactional approach in terms of improved task performance, social support, and perceived effectiveness, and lower negative affect. Therefore, the rigidity of the rules and guidelines of the transactional leadership style can prevent workers from engaging with each other socially and, in extreme cases, drive workers toward mobilization and immobilization. This could be a source of increased stress and burnout in healthcare organizations that rely heavily on a transactional leadership approach that ignores the human element.

The Benefits and Drawbacks of Transactional Leadership

Transactional leadership has several strengths and weaknesses compared to other leadership styles. Foremost, the approach gained a significant reputation because it relies on tried-and-tested organizational strategies to lead employees and induce commitment (Potter and Starcke 2022). Although the benefits can be amplified by combining it with the transformational style, transactional leadership is highly favorable because it is supported by considerable evidence and promotes favorable individual and organizational outcomes. The second benefit stems from its emphasis on contingent-based reward systems. This term implies that an organization relies on incentive-based structures that are tied to the behavior and performance of employees. Accordingly, employees are rewarded if they meet predetermined outcomes and expectations. For that reason, these rewards often appeal to the followers' self-interest by encouraging them to pursue the best rewards. These factors explain the high popularity of the transactional leadership style in modern organizations as a strategy for guiding decision-making and stimulating productivity.

With regard to its drawbacks, the transactional leadership has been criticized due to its outcomes and lack of personal identification. Foremost, the transactional approach encourages workers to deliver high levels of returns, but this often results in predictable outcomes instead of outstanding performance. While this leadership style is designed to strengthen organizational productivity, workers are usually driven to pursue acceptable levels of return instead of performing to their fullest potential. As a result, this weakness can negatively affect an organization's productivity. For example, healthcare workers are frequently asked to see more patients and submit more billable services each workday. If an organization pushes too strongly and neglects stress levels in their workforce, employees may end up reverting back to doing the bare minimum.

Self-actualization is often neglected in this leadership style, which can easily result in job dissatisfaction. Without intrinsic motivation, it can be difficult to interact with employees on a personal level, while at the same time creating a poor environment for social engagement. Regarding personal identification, the transactional approach places little emphasis on the employees' self-esteem. The lack of personal identification between leaders and subordinates often results in an unequal distribution of power between them. This problem can weaken the relationships between the leader and the followers (Odumeru and Ogbonna 2013). Overall, the declining use of the transactional leadership style can be attributed to its predictable outcomes and the lack of emphasis on intrinsic motivation.

> **Case Study 4.1: Providing Structure**
>
> At Safe Haven Medical Clinic, Dr. Cole realizes that transactional leadership is appropriate given the immediate challenge of unprecedented surges in patient numbers, increased workload, and emotional toll. The transactional leadership style, characterized by a structured chain of command, rewards (e.g., being given preferred schedules, extra time off, or perks such as meals), and punishments (e.g., frequent reminders to work harder and less autonomy over schedule), aligns with the need for a clear organizational structure and efficient task management.
>
> Given the urgency of the situation, Dr. Cole can use transactional leadership to provide a framework for addressing immediate concerns, such as task delegation, adherence to rules and regulations, and rewarding healthcare workers for their efforts. The focus on extrinsic motivation – including recognition, support, and perks such as extra time off, access to more preferred schedules, and financial support for continuing education – can serve as a timely reinforcement to boost morale and engagement. In the face of rising stress levels and potential resignations, transactional leadership offers a methodical approach to managing the workforce and ensuring that tasks are completed efficiently.
>
> However, it's crucial for Dr. Cole to balance transactional leadership with an awareness of its potential drawbacks, such as the risk of increased stress and anxiety among workers due to the rigid structure and lack of emphasis on intrinsic motivation. While transactional leadership may address immediate challenges, Dr. Cole should also consider incorporating elements of other leadership styles, such as transformational or servant leadership, to foster long-term employee well-being and satisfaction.

Transformational Leadership

The transformational leadership style is the opposite of transactional leadership. In essence, this approach requires leaders to inspire their followers to think beyond their immediate self-interests. This goal can be achieved through idealized influence, charisma, and intellectual stimulation (Khan et al. 2020). This explains why the transformational leadership style is considered the opposite of transactional leadership. Its emphasis on intrinsic and extrinsic motivation implies that it is a suitable leadership approach for visionary leaders who want to rally their staff to support the organization's vision. Transformational leaders often dedicate significant amounts of time and effort toward inspiring their followers to align with the organization's core values, including improving health outcomes and customer satisfaction, as well as hopefully reducing costs and unintended negative outcomes (complications). Examples in healthcare include the charge nurse who actively helps out on the floor and supports the nursing staff, and the hospital executive who takes time to sit with employees and make themselves available to troubleshoot and obtain feedback from those on the front lines.

A major characteristic of transformational leadership is its ability to create a good match between an organization's activities and employees' behaviors and values. Recent research reveals that transformational leaders place considerable focus on acquiring the employees' recognition based on their competencies, strengths, and weaknesses (Choi et al. 2016). This approach allows the leader to create solid relationships with their subordinates. If the leader succeeds in becoming a role model, they will be in an ideal position to positively influence the team, stimulating them to reach their full potential. In addition, transformational leaders often highlight creativity and innovation when solving problems and improving organizational outcomes during times of uncertainty.

While these findings do not shed light on whether transformational leadership is superior to transactional leadership, they highlight its alignment with the social engagement (ventral vagal) state of the PVT. At its core, the social engagement state is about feeling safe and connected. Transformational leaders usually perform actions that inspire their followers. As a result, this sense of shared vision and values encourages social engagement and contributes to a more engaging workplace. In the social engagement state, open communication channels and trust can strengthen workers' feelings of safety, thereby encouraging workers to perform optimally.

The Benefits and Drawbacks of Transformational Leadership

The transformational leadership style has a wide variety of strengths and weaknesses. The most evident advantage of the transformational leadership style lies in its dual focus on organizational performance and employee well-being. Research reveals that there is a direct relationship between transformational leadership and optimized organizational performance (Khan et al. 2020). Compared to the transactional leadership style, which neglects employees' intrinsic motivation, transformational leadership focuses on employees' holistic well-being.

In addition, this leadership style also promotes creativity and innovation by encouraging workers to "think outside the box." For example, employees may innovate more efficient ways to process admissions and discharges of patients from their hospital unit. Fundamentally, the transformational leadership approach inspires workers to be open-minded and embrace diverse ideas. As a result, this benefit is essential for augmenting organizational productivity. The final benefit relates to the style's ability to create strong teams. This leadership style encourages leaders to monitor their subordinates while simultaneously creating opportunities for the exchange of ideas and skills between the workers. As a result, the transformational leadership approach is highly suitable for building strong relationships and fostering a sense of unity among team members.

The main weakness of this style stems from its high dependency on the leader for decision-making. In most cases, the leader is portrayed as the role model, so situations may arise where the leader is considered the workers' only source of guidance and inspiration. In such situations, followers may struggle to take the initiative without direct support from the leader. Another drawback is that the transformational leadership style prioritizes idealized influence over group-level processes and interactions (Jensen et al. 2016). In other words, most transformational leaders prioritize the well-being of individual employees, but neglect consideration of external factors such as stakeholder engagement and resource management. Transformational leadership has also been criticized due to the lack of clarity in its definition and characteristics (Banks et al. 2016). The concept of transformational leadership is quite broad; thus, there is considerable uncertainty concerning its practical applications in real-life scenarios, including the more highly structured healthcare services that rely on established workflows, algorithms, and high levels of acuity. Hence, the transformational leadership style can be criticized for its overdependency on leaders, its tendency to neglect group-level factors, and its ambiguity.

> **Case Study 4.2: Transforming the Workplace**
>
> Dr. Cole is grappling with increasing stress levels and potential resignations among the staff at Safe Haven Medical Clinic. The current situation demands a leadership style that goes beyond the traditional transactional approach, which might be contributing to stress and dissatisfaction. Transformational leadership is particularly relevant in this context because it emphasizes inspiring and motivating the staff to work beyond their personal interests. Given the high-pressure environment, transformational leadership can help Dr. Cole foster a sense of shared vision and values and promote open communication channels. As a transformational leader, Dr. Cole needs to dedicate significant time and effort to inspire the staff to align with the clinic's core values.
>
> Adopting a transformational leadership style allows Dr. Cole to not only alleviate stress levels among healthcare workers but also to foster a more resilient and committed workforce capable of dealing with the rising patient demands. However, Dr. Cole should also be mindful of potential drawbacks of the transformational leadership style, such as the high dependency on her for decision-making and the need to balance individual well-being with broader organizational considerations. Still, transformational leadership is strongly associated with safety, which is a crucial factor for activating the social engagement system and keeping her staff satisfied and motivated.

Situational Leadership

The situational leadership style has been embraced as an innovative leadership style for healthcare workers because it allows leaders to adjust their strategies in accordance with the emerging situation. In the early days, researchers developed the idea that situational leadership can be nurtured by allocating enough time and resources to strengthen the leader's traits. As a result, situational leadership was developed with the primary objective of creating a solid structure for guiding leaders across the various leadership styles in a flexible way (Ghazzawi et al. 2017).

Nowadays, situational leadership largely depends on the leader's ability to diagnose situational conditions and initiate prompt responses to emerging issues. Accordingly, this leadership is based on three key principles: (1) the amount of direction and guidance a leader can provide, (2) the amount of social and emotional support a leader can provide, and (3) the worker's capability to perform a specific task. Given that healthcare environments are often highly unpredictable, situational leadership allows leaders to adjust their styles to address the circumstances they are facing.

Furthermore, situational leadership emphasizes the importance of considering the experience levels of an organization's workers. Thompson and Glasø (2018) explain that leaders can use directiveness to handle new employees, and then gradually shift to more supportive strategies as the workers become more familiar with their roles and responsibilities. Initially, situational leaders often take on a directive role by providing guidance and direction to workers. This goal emerges because new employees often demand more explicit guidance as compared to seasoned workers. Therefore, as the employees gain adequate knowledge and skills, the need for direct support decreases. This change allows the situational leader to be more supportive in terms of providing encouragement and promoting their autonomy. In this context, effective leadership should be adaptable to the needs of both new and well-seasoned workers to improve its outcomes.

Situational leadership requires leaders who can shift between the different autonomic states set forth by the PVT. This shift has been compared to climbing up and down the polyvagal ladder (see Chapter 1: "What is the Polyvagal Ladder"). At the beginning of their leadership journeys, these leaders need to be active and responsive to emerging issues, such as indoctrinating new workers. Similarly, a fundamental component of the PVT is its emphasis on having the ability to respond to environmental cues and recognize potential stressors. Furthermore, although situational leadership is not oriented toward stress, it can allow leaders to moderate their stress levels by providing direction or support depending on the workers' experience and skill levels.

Benefits and Drawbacks of Situational Leadership

Although the situational leadership style is still relatively new, it has several evident strengths and weaknesses. For instance, it is particularly effective in training and academic settings (Thompson and Glasø 2018). This benefit emerges because the style is designed to take into consideration the skills and knowledge of employees across their career path. For that reason, situational leadership is highly recommended for leaders who prioritize the growth and well-being of their workers in the long term. This strength revolves around the idea that different employees require different types of leadership depending on their skill and experience levels.

In addition, situational leadership provides an easy-to-follow framework for explaining how leaders should respond to different organizational needs, such as balancing customer experience with managing demands on fast, efficient care, while navigating payor and regulatory expectations. By tailoring the leadership to the readiness and competence of the team members, it is possible to enhance employee engagement and their overall performance. Considering that situational leadership is relatively effective in training settings, and it can be easily implemented, this style may offer significant rewards in healthcare settings. These could include increased job satisfaction, decreased levels of stress, and enhanced ventral vagal socialization due to cues of safety (as employees see their skills being acknowledged appropriately).

Despite the benefits, some researchers argue that evidence for the real-life application of this leadership approach is lacking. This problem is compounded by the fact that the definition of this style has undergone numerous revisions to refine its concepts and practicality, which has served only to increase its complexity. Another major challenge concerning situational leadership is that it places too great a burden on the leaders. Although adaptability is a crucial trait in any organization, there is no certainty that leaders can demonstrate the right levels of flexibility in every situation, particularly in high-stress environments.

This leadership style places more emphasis on adaptable leadership over decision-making, so it can be quite challenging for navigating complex situations. Overall, the high level of uncertainty surrounding situational leadership hinders its application in many organizations. In healthcare settings, the correct decision in patient care may not always be readily apparent, and situations can be somewhat unpredictable. In an effort to be too flexible, this can cause confusion and uncertainty.

> **Case Study 4.3: Facing the Surge Flexibly**
>
> As mentioned, the surge of incoming patients has led to heightened stress among the workers. In this high-pressure scenario, the situational leadership style can be a valuable framework for Dr. Cole to tailor her leadership approach based on the specific requirements and maturity levels of the workforce.
>
> Given the unpredictable nature of the environment and the diverse levels of experience among the staff, situational leadership empowers Dr. Cole to assess situational conditions promptly and to respond effectively to emerging challenges. As healthcare workers acquire knowledge and skills or become more acquainted with their roles, situational leadership advocates for a transition toward more supportive strategies, fostering autonomy and providing encouragement. In this context, Dr. Cole may initially assume a more directive role, offering explicit guidance and support, particularly for newer employees who require clearer direction.
>
> However, if Dr. Cole fails to implement situational leadership effectively, the drawbacks can easily outweigh the benefits. Given the complexity of healthcare settings and the varying levels of experience among the staff, situational leadership requires her to find a delicate balance. Without this balance, Dr. Cole may overburden herself while dealing with various problems. This dynamic nature of the healthcare environment is a major concern that needs to be taken into consideration when implementing situational leadership. Otherwise, this leadership style can demonstrate significant results in terms of alleviating work-related stress at Safe Haven and improving employee satisfaction.

Servant Leadership

Compared to transactional and transformational leaders, which have long histories, the servant leadership style is relatively new. This style encourages leaders to prioritize the well-being of their workers rather than pursue organizational benefits or personal glory. Contrary to common misconceptions, servant leadership does not imply that the leader should be subservient to their followers. Instead, leaders are required to inspire their followers by appealing to their personal values and virtues; they exercise their power and authority with the aim of enhancing their followers' autonomy (Winston and Fields 2015). In addition, they also dedicate significant time to interacting with, educating, and inspiring their subordinates, with the ultimate objective of encouraging them to reach their full potential. In a healthcare setting, we often see this in educational institutions that provide intensive mentoring and support for trainees in medicine and nursing. Additionally, some clinical services may utilize highly skilled senior staff to mentor and support junior members, as in a traditional apprenticeship model.

The main aspect of servant leadership lies in the leader's commitment to altruistic motives and creating a positive organizational culture through spirituality. In the workplace, spirituality defines the workers' acknowledgment of their inner values and beliefs. It does not merely describe a person's adherence to specific religious convictions, but, rather, acknowledges the importance of following particular principles. In healthcare, this ties in with values around human dignity, serving those who are suffering and providing support to patients at very vulnerable times of their lives. The servant leader will model this focus on helping others. With that said, the interactions between the servant leader and the followers are usually oriented toward strengthening the collaboration between different workers. Therefore, servant leadership places a lot of attention on building trust and on shared decision-making, instead of relying on self-serving and opportunistic leadership styles (Whittington 2017). The most evident distinction of servant leadership lies in its objective of selflessly serving one's subordinates to inspire them to deliver optimal performance.

Similar to the transformational leadership style, servant leadership is also closely aligned with the social engagement state of the PVT. In essence, servant leaders usually prioritize creating a trusting and safe environment for their followers through transparency, open communication, and genuinely caring about the needs and concerns of their team members. They also highlight the importance of empowering workers through shared decision-making. This empowerment coincides with the social engagement (ventral vagal) state's focus on being in control of one's actions and creating safe social environments. Trust is inherent to the social engagement state because it allows workers to feel secure and fosters positive social interactions. As a result, the servant leadership approach can be employed by leaders who desire to remain in the social engagement state of the ANS.

The Benefits and Drawbacks of Servant Leadership

Servant leadership is a less common leadership style compared to the transformational, transactional, and situational approaches. However, it has gained a lot of traction in recent years. According to Specchia et al. (2021), servant leadership can play a major role in optimizing an organization's performance by integrating different professional competencies, including teamwork, collective decision-making, and ethics. As such, this leadership style can create an organizational culture that is built on trust and ethical behaviors.

In transactional and transformation leadership approaches, the underlying focus is on the workers' intrinsic and extrinsic motivation. Contrarily, servant leadership is simpler because it does not depend on remunerating the workers. This explains why servant leadership is one of the least complicated leadership strategies. Despite its simplicity, servant leaders can easily navigate change because they often have their employees' support. By empowering their workers, these leaders can gain the favor of their employees, thereby cultivating a healthy workforce.

With regard to weaknesses, servant leadership has several critical flaws. For instance, the leader is required to sacrifice personal rewards and advancement to improve staff productivity and overall organizational performance. Although servant leadership is a noble style, in reality it is impractical in many organizations. Very few leaders are willing to sacrifice their rewards and benefits for their followers. For example, a physician who spends most of their time mentoring others and solving staff issues is less available for direct patient care and billable services, thereby reducing their revenue significantly. In addition, the leadership style is surrounded by a lot of uncertainty. Furthermore, there is a high likelihood that the employees will take advantage of their leaders' willingness to serve them, resulting in a reduction in their accountability. Winston and Fields (2015) explain that there is very little consensus among researchers concerning the real-life applications of servant leadership. Existing research on this leadership style reveals that there are discrepancies concerning the need for trust, love, humility, wisdom, healing, and spirituality (Winston and Fields 2015). In addition, this style can hinder decision-making because shared decision-making is often slower than when a single person makes decisions. Therefore, these drawbacks can prevent healthcare organizations and individual leaders from adopting the servant leadership style. However, some elements of servant leadership may be used in situations to further support employees and staff.

> **Case Study 4.4: Becoming the Servant Leader**
>
> Dr. Cole believes that the servant leadership style, which prioritizes the well-being of the workers over the leader's self-interests, is a suitable approach for dealing with the current issues at Safe Haven Medical Clinic. The style's focus on altruistic motives and fostering collaboration resonates with the need for transparency, open communication, and genuine care about the needs and concerns of healthcare professionals. Understanding that trust is the bedrock of effective teamwork and collaboration, Dr. Cole prioritizes transparency and shows a genuine concern for the needs and concerns of the clinic's staff. By actively cultivating trust within the organizational framework, Dr. Cole aims to create an environment wherein individuals feel secure, supported, and motivated to contribute their best efforts.
>
> Nonetheless, while the servant leadership style offers benefits such as trust-building, ethical behavior, and a positive organizational culture, Dr. Cole knows she must be mindful of potential drawbacks, including the sacrifice required from leaders and the risk of reduced accountability among employees. However, in the context of a healthcare setting where the well-being of healthcare workers is crucial for optimal patient care, servant leadership's emphasis on supporting and empowering employees may prove to be a valuable and relevant leadership style.

Embracing Steadfast Leadership

Steadfast leadership is a form of leadership that we used in our prior book (Brazie and Vanderpal 2023), which emerges from the balance between rational (cognitive) and nonrational (intuitive) decision-making faculties. While many researchers emphasize the importance of intelligence quotient (IQ) and rational decision-making, the reality is that emotional quotient (EQ) and nonrational decision-making are equally important.

In most cases, EQ and nonrational faculties are often viewed as impediments to optimal decision-making. However, neuroscience shows that EQ is strongly associated with the neural components that evaluate risks and rewards. Research reveals that the emotional and cognitive process of the human body are intertwined, and this integration strongly influences risk behavior. Based on neural imaging, several sections of the brain involved in emotional processing (the anterior insula, amygdala, and the ventromedial prefrontal cortex) are crucial for activating risk responses (Sánchez-López et al. 2022). Considering that emotional stimuli are an inherent aspect of being human, leaders need to recognize their importance in decision-making. Striking an equilibrium between rational and nonrational decision-making can allow leaders to harness different cognitive faculties, allowing them to make better leadership decisions. This approach not only acknowledges the undeniable impact of emotions on decision-making, but also leverages them strategically to optimize an organization's outcomes. Specifically for healthcare organizations, we have touched upon measures such as stress and burnout in staff, patient satisfaction, and clinical outcomes. Other measures that should be positively impacted by an instinctive leadership approach include length of stay (the shorter the better), less rapid readmissions within 30 days, and decreased visits to emergency rooms after discharge.

Leaders need to understand their employees in order to lead workers and drive them to perform to their full potential. *Intuition* can be defined as a decision-making mechanism that relies on a person's ability to make rapid and nonconscious judgments by recognizing patterns and associations. In other words, intuition relies on a person's ability to develop gut instincts using existing knowledge. The field of neuroscience has begun to place considerable emphasis on intuition and instinctive decision-making because they are becoming more crucial when addressing urgent clinical matters and supervising healthcare workers, especially during periods of high demand. That said, steadfast leadership is essential for encouraging leaders to be more conscious of their workers' emotions and minds in order to make optimal choices. A unique challenge in HR matters is trying to balance providing cues of safety with needing to follow consistent, predictable policies that may take more time to properly follow. This means that not all decisions should be made rapidly, depending on the situation.

The inadequacy of research regarding intuitive decision-making is a critical research gap in the healthcare sector. Bacon (2013, 1) asks the following questions about intuitive leadership: "Can you think of an occasion where you've had a gut feeling that something wasn't right about a significant business issue but didn't listen to your intuition and later regretted it? Do you often doubt your intuition in favor of hard evidence to support your business decisions?" If the answer is yes, then there is a high likelihood that the individual is underutilizing one of their most powerful mental faculties – intuitive intelligence.

According to Bacon, intuition is more than a gut feeling because it is based on a person's ability to piece together information using data from their surroundings, experiences, or options (Bacon 2013). To sum up, the journey to cultivating steadfast leadership in the healthcare industry begins with embracing the benefits of rational and nonrational faculties when making decisions. This does not mean that healthcare leaders should act prematurely in the absence of sufficient information and consideration. Rather, we see the benefits of understanding emotions and how they are impacted by the nervous system state on the polyvagal ladder. By combining verbal and nonverbal skills, a steadfast healthcare leader can provide guidance, support, and structure as the organization navigates complex clinical, regulatory, and business needs.

Ultimately, by using a balance of rational and nonrational approaches, the healthcare leader can consider each of the leadership styles discussed and make a decision on which of these is appropriate in each situation. As mentioned, in high-acuity situations involving emergencies, surgical procedures, or intensive care, there is a need for a more structured, transactional approach. Outpatient clinics, especially in behavioral health, may find a servant and/or transformational leadership approach the most helpful.

> **Case Study 4.5: Using Steadfast Leadership**
>
> Dr. Jennings and Dr. Cole often face problems involving high patient influxes and low employee satisfaction at Safe Haven Clinic. As a result, they have a basic understanding of the root causes of such situations and the necessary steps that should be taken in response. Therefore, steadfast leadership begins with Dr. Cole acknowledging the importance of her intuition and emotional intelligence. Intuitive decision-making requires her to look for patterns in her knowledge base to make more balanced decisions involving her employees' emotional responses, as well as carefully monitoring her own polyvagal state and avoiding acting on biases.
>
> By recognizing the value of the rational and nonrational sides of her decision-making faculty, she will have a more solid understanding of the reasons why her best workers are considering resigning. With steadfast leadership, she can incorporate the leadership style that her organization requires, allowing her to shift between the transactional, transformational, servant, and situational styles when necessary. In the end, steadfast leadership can prompt a healthcare leader toward success by driving them to embrace rational and nonrational cognitive processes.

Common Characteristics of Good Leaders

Recent breakthroughs in neuroscience have highlighted the existence of a "social brain network": a collection of brain areas that function together to allow people to interact with others (Platt 2020). This social brain gives human beings the ability to objectively identify members of society with strong leadership skills and those who would benefit from skill improvement, as well as which interventions have the highest likelihood of paying off.

In 2008, Google began Project Oxygen, which aimed to determine what makes a great manager (Platt 2020). The project uncovered the most crucial traits for leaders who desire improvement in organizational outcomes, such as turnover, satisfaction, and performance. These eight traits are (1) good coaching, (2) empowering team members, (3) expressing personal interest in the members' well-being, (4) having a result-oriented mentality, (5) good communication, (6) supporting employees with career development, (7) having a clear vision and strategy, and (8) having key technical skills. Neuroscientific research suggest that such leadership traits *can* be cultivated. These traits suggest a style more along the lines of transformational, servant, and even situational leadership.

In all cases, successful leadership requires a person to have a highly attuned ANS – that is, to be someone who can easily shift between socialization (ventral vagal state) and mobilization (sympathetic state) as needed to optimize decision-making. Specific traits identified for good decision-making include judgment, courage, accountability, justice, integrity, humility, humanity, collaboration, and drive (Seijts and Gandz 2018). These traits can strengthen the leader's approach in both the social engagement and mobilization states. Nonetheless, each trait is generally oriented toward a specific function. For example, courage drives leaders to confront challenging situations, while justice and integrity are vital for making ethical and morally appropriate decisions. Among these traits, good judgment has been cited as the most useful trait, followed by courage (Seijts and Gandz 2018).

> **Team Chemistry**
>
> Most organizations acknowledge the importance of selecting team members with a good fit to optimize the organization's outcomes. Neuroscience research reveals that "team chemistry" is a real-life concept that emerges due to synchronization between the team members. In essence, team chemistry describes how well the ventral vagal socialization state is functioning among team members. As we have discussed, this involves communication, emotion, and bodily reactions as workers interact with one another. As workers feel safe and supported, they are able to connect with one another and become more creative and productive. In the early 2000s, researchers identified that strong teams have compelling direction, a strong structure, and a supportive context. However, they also discovered a fourth facet – shared mindset – which fosters a common understanding between the individual members.
>
> A significant issue facing teams today involves the tendency of leaders to put together teams without considering the interplay of the chemistry or traits between the individual members. Taking these findings into consideration, healthcare leaders need to recognize the importance of team chemistry when establishing and leading teams. Methods to enhance team chemistry include providing cues of safety in communications, encouraging team-building exercises, and actively coaching team members to support and encourage one another.

Polyvagal-Informed Strategies for Leading in High-Stress Environments

A team is made up of individuals who each have a dominant polyvagal state. From there, each worker will usually shift among the three polyvagal states throughout the day, depending on the surrounding circumstances. As you might assume, most workers in high-stress environments are SNS dominant (mobilized and at the ready). This can be helpful in healthcare settings where many patients must be attended to promptly and efficiently; however, without ventral vagal regulation, those who maintain a high level of mobilization are in danger of burnout (the dorsal vagal state).

The ideal is for healthcare workers to function, even under pressure, from a ventral vagal state with enough mobilization from their SNS to attend to their duties and provide appropriate healthcare to patients. Fortunately, it is relatively easy to help workers shift out of a flight-or-fight response with various polyvagal-informed strategies. Teach, demonstrate, and encourage ANS regulation throughout the workers' shifts.

On-the-Go Polyvagal Skills for High-Stress Environments

Workers in high-stress environments are often so engaged with their outer needs that they have difficulty spending sufficient time maintaining inward focus to reap immediate benefits. Sharing the polyvagal-informed exercises in Chapter 1 with the staff through targeted meetings and workshops can give them the skills to regulate their ANS, but quick, on-the-go tools can also be taught easily and quickly for awareness.

One of the best things about these tools is that they can take only a few seconds or a few minutes to reduce stress or burnout. When practiced often, you and your staff can improve your performance, mood, and quality of life. Here are a few techniques to use and teach:

- **Find the "moments between."** Bring your awareness to the seconds between actions. For example, sense your feet grounded on the floor when sitting or as you walk across the room. Orient yourself by noticing sensory qualities of the station or room you are in before moving on. Silently name what you have accomplished *before* you go to the next task.
- **Spend a moment "seeing" others.** Rather than shifting your eyes away from others that you pass by during the course of your day, make a conscious effort to notice them. In a recent study, nurses were asked to gather between shifts. Those clocking out were asked to raise their hands, and those clocking in would look at them. This allowed the nurses to see there was an ending to their shifts. Over time the nurses reported that this simple practice helped them to feel more connected with their coworkers and they noticed lower stress levels. It was also designed to increase moments of ventral vagal state whenever the staff was gathered in meetings (Flarity, Gentry, and Mesnikoft 2013).
- **Notice more "transitional movement."** Identify your polyvagal state when you transition from one location to the next. For example, when you get into your car to head to work, take a moment to identify your state and regulate it as needed, perhaps with a breathing exercise. As you exit your car, notice again. Quickly self-reference your internal state with each new location.
- **Simple tactile orienting.** Become aware of something you are touching. This does not take away from anything you are doing in the moment. For example, if your arms are crossed, you might feel the fabric of your clothing. If your hands are on a tabletop, you may notice a cool or hard sensation.
- **Create a sense of personal containment.** The way you stand or sit can offer you a sense of personal safety by creating a boundary between yourself and another whose ANS may be dysregulated. For example, place your hands together or cross your arms or legs. A side benefit of crossing your legs and tuning into your interoceptive sensations is a feeling of being grounded.

ANS Regulation Script for Group Meetings

Meetings are a routine daily occurrence in most healthcare settings, whether it be clinical patient rounds or administrative functions. When done thoughtfully, modeling good ventral vagal socialization in each meeting is an excellent opportunity to build connection and cohesion. Ideally, those who are leading the meetings will take time beforehand to check their own nervous system state on the polyvagal ladder and make efforts to move out of immobilization or excess mobilization before leading others. This will help the others in the room to either remain in or shift to a more socialized state.

Typically, in most meetings leaders allow a couple of minutes or so for all attendees to arrive and settle. The following are step-by-step examples of how one could demonstrate and promote regulation skills in a group setting.

1. *Once everyone is settled:* "Before we begin, let's take a moment to look around. Notice where you are sitting and who is near you. Take a few moments to connect to the person on each side of you." *After two minutes, the meeting proceeds.*
2. *Following the initial presentation:* "Before we go on, let's take a moment to stretch; stand up if you'd like." *After one minute:* "Does anyone feel more present than they did before?" *Respond to any answers. The meeting proceeds.*
3. *If the meeting becomes heated or feels rushed:* "This conversation has sped up. I'd like to remind everyone of their polyvagal tools. Let's all take a moment to consciously slow down."
4. *If the meeting lacks luster and eyes are closing:* "If you're disconnecting, bring yourself back. If you're falling asleep, engage your muscles and bring some clarity back."
5. *To engage wandering attention:* "Hey, has anyone noticed..." *(talk about something everyone will look at).*
6. *If disagreements are interfering with the productivity of the meeting:* "Everyone stand up. Think about something you stand for. Let yourself really sense into that. Now look around the room. People are standing up for change in the world. We may have different ways of doing that. Society needs that – many ways to solve common issues. Now let's return to our common goal for this meeting. Everyone here is working toward that similar goal."

When it comes time for the meeting to adjourn, leaders can ensure they make eye contact with the attendees and verbalize the closing. Some leaders enjoy inviting members to stand and move, while others may use lighthearted humor or a fun story to close in a highly socialized way. Additionally, some type of summary or action points to take up before the next meeting may be communicated prior to final closing. Be sure to keep things in a socialization state, though you can also invite some mild SNS play by introducing health mobilization that maintains connection between individuals. This helps the group to disperse and go about their day with a sense of well-being and confidence.

Stress-Management Interventions

The most effective approach for creating a conducive work environment is to embrace a variety of stress-management interventions. From the polyvagal perspective, these interventions not only focus on addressing the psychological and emotional aspects, but also modulate the ANS to be more resilient to stress. Such interventions are particularly essential for healthcare workers, who often work in demanding and high-pressure situations.

In essence, there are three categories of stress-management interventions: primary, secondary, and tertiary. According to Bhui et al. (2016), primary interventions strive to address the causal factors of stress, whereas secondary interventions aim to reduce the duration or severity of symptoms. In other words, primary interventions prioritize reducing and minimizing a person's exposure to stressors, whereas secondary measures strive to support the safe response to and management of stress symptoms once they emerge following a crisis. Last, tertiary interventions are designed to enable a person to maximize their functionality through rehabilitation. Compared to primary and secondary interventions, tertiary mechanisms aim to revitalize a person to full recovery. These three approaches provide a holistic strategy for mitigating trauma and stress in accordance with the PVT, as illustrated in Figure 4.3.

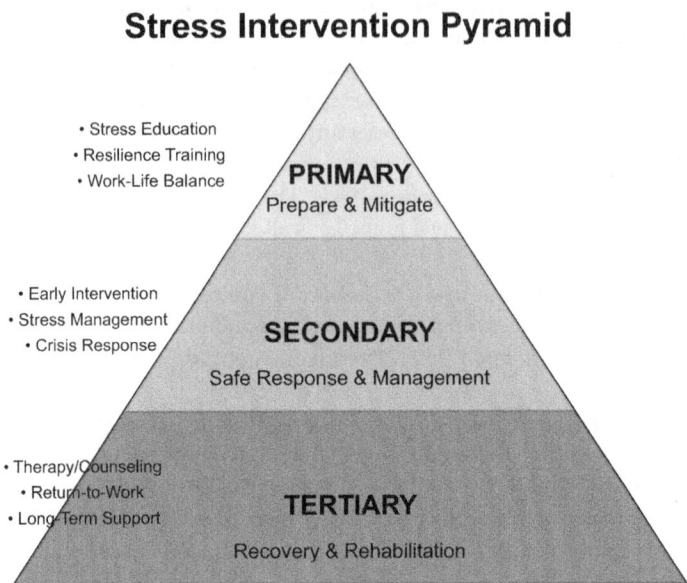

Figure 4.3 Primary, secondary, and tertiary stress interventions. (Source: authors.)

Primary Interventions

Primary interventions usually focus on addressing the underlying cause of stress by promoting a physiological state that is conducive to emotional regulation and resilience. These approaches stem from the idea that stress is the consequence of a lack of fit between the demands on and the needs of healthcare workers. Accordingly, primary interventions focus on adapting to the environment to create a better fit with the individual. For instance, the physical and mental demands should be commensurate with the workers' capabilities and resources. This approach involves making provisions to allow healthcare workers to recover when handling demanding tasks. With regard to work schedules, the organization should ensure that the schedules are conducive so that the workers do not need to work beyond their official work hours. A suitable recommendation is to use rotating shifts to create more structure in the work schedule.

In addition, there should be clarity in terms of promotion and skill development to create a sense of safety within the workforce. Creating this sense of safety can play a vital role in increasing job satisfaction and reducing employee turnover. The social environment should also be favorable in terms of personal interactions and emotional support. Many organizations ignore the social factor because it does not bring tangible benefits to performance, but social interactions can make work more engaging.

The final primary intervention involves designing job tasks so that they have meaning and stimulate the employees. This goal can be achieved by job rotation or increasing the scope of work activities. Primary interventions can be considered a vehicle for culture change because the type of action required by the organization will depend on the stressors causing the problem. Although clinical service needs may render some of these interventions difficult to implement in healthcare settings at times (e.g., when demand is overloading capacity), they are vital for emotional regulation and resilience.

Secondary Interventions

Secondary interventions aim to reduce the hypervigilance of the ANS, thereby reducing the severity and duration of stress symptoms. These interventions are primarily concerned with the prompt detection and management of the stress experienced by the worker (Bhui et al. 2016).

There are many individual factors that affect how employees respond to stress or perceived threats. Considering that there are workers who can tolerate working in high-pressure healthcare environments and those who cannot suggests that people tolerate different levels of stress. This threshold can vary depending on the person's behavioral response, the situation, their age, or experiences. In this context, secondary preventions include stress education and stress management. For example, healthcare workers can try relaxation training, cognitive coping skills, or lifestyle modification. Compared to primary interventions, these recommendations focus on helping the individual cope with organizational situations that cannot be altered. As such, the most crucial aspect of secondary interventions lies in their goal of limiting damage by addressing the consequences of the stressors, rather than dealing with the sources of stress. To sum up, secondary interventions can be considered the "Band-Aid" of stress management.

Tertiary Interventions

These interventions focus on rehabilitation and maximizing functioning by fostering a sense of safety and social connectedness, which is crucial in regulating the ANS. These interventions are primarily concerned with rehabilitation and improving recovery, especially among individuals with serious health complications caused by stress. Accordingly, these interventions are specialized for improving a healthcare worker's ability to deal with chronic stress levels.

In healthcare organizations, tertiary interventions occur through employee counseling and employee assistance programs. These programs are designed so that employees can be referred to appropriate treatment facilities if they demonstrate that they are unable to cope with their stressors. In most cases, employees can volunteer to go for counseling and return to work after a period of time. Counseling is an evidence-based approach to improving the psychological well-being of workers. Healthcare workers who work in high-stress situations need to embrace these interventions if they want to recover and return to work at full capacity.

Stress-management interventions can play a vital role in reducing burnout among healthcare workers by providing them with the right tools to cope with the stresses and the emotional demands of their profession. As a result, it is possible to increase workers' levels of concentration, satisfaction, and performance. Furthermore, the right stress-management intervention can indirectly benefit patients by ensuring that healthcare workers are mentally and emotionally equipped to deliver appropriate care. Although these interventions may require workers to collaborate in team settings, these groups play a major role in building supportive and cohesive work environments. The ultimate objective is to build a resilient workforce that can thrive when faced with adversity and bounce back from challenging situations. In learning about the PVT and implementing the tools discussed in this book, we hope healthcare leaders and workers will be armed with new skills and greater understanding to help them navigate their daily work lives.

> **Case Study 4.6: Managing Stress**
>
> The problems identified at Safe Haven Clinic largely stem from excessive stress in the workplace. Accordingly, the three stress-management strategies noted herein can be employed in sequence to mitigate stress and its impact at the facility. Primary stress-management interventions target the underlying cause of stress by altering the work environment to match the individual's needs and capabilities. This intervention can be applied by restructuring work schedules to provide recovery time, clarifying skill requirements and responsibilities, and creating a more positive social environment.
>
> Secondary interventions may be integrated to manage workers' stress symptoms and improve the detection of such events. Dr. Cole can encourage the workers to participate in stress-education activities, relaxation training, and lifestyle modification to reduce their stress levels. Tertiary interventions that focus on rehabilitation and maximizing the workers' function can be introduced to provide long-term support to the workers. Examples of such activities include employee assistance and counseling programs.
>
> While Safe Haven may struggle to implement the three categories of responses, it should ensure that there is a specific intervention designed for preparedness, mitigation, response, and recovery. The PVT helps in understanding how the human nervous system responds and how we may assist others in shifting back into a more ventral vagal state of socialization and safety.

Key Takeaways

- The healthcare sector's inherent exposure to stress and trauma has profound implications for the well-being of healthcare workers. The prevalence of high stress levels underscores the urgency for proactive strategies to support these professionals. While a significant proportion of healthcare workers exhibit resilience to stress and trauma, there is a substantial minority facing adverse psychological and behavioral outcomes. Distress reactions, psychiatric disorders, and high-risk behaviors can pose long-term health risks. Recognizing these outcomes is essential for healthcare organizations to prioritize the mental and physical well-being of their workforce and mitigate the detrimental effects of consistent exposure to stress and trauma. Overall, a holistic approach to employee well-being is imperative, encompassing preventive measures, mental health support, and interventions tailored to individual needs.
- The historical evolution of leadership reflects the intricate interplay of innate traits and nurtured skills. The identified leadership styles offer distinctive approaches with inherent strengths and weaknesses. Foremost, transactional leadership provides reliability and efficiency but risks stifling intrinsic motivation and hindering social engagement. In comparison, transformational leadership aligns with the PVT's social engagement state but may face challenges in decision-making distribution and clarity. Meanwhile, situational leadership is adaptive and responsive, but demands a delicate balance and may excessively burden leaders. Last, servant leadership prioritizes the employees' well-being and also resonates with the PVT's emphasis on safety and trust, but requires leaders to sacrifice personal benefits. Ultimately, the most effective leadership style for healthcare professionals may involve a judicious blend of these approaches, using steadfast leadership as the foundation to ensure an optimal polyvagal state.

- Building strong teams that perform efficiently in high-stress environments requires a comprehensive understanding of the characteristics essential for both team leaders and team members. Effective team leadership involves a combination of strategies: coaching, empowerment, personal engagement, results orientation, communication, career support, strategic vision, and technical proficiency. There are also specific traits that leaders should strive to nurture, with good judgment and courage being assigned the highest priority. Moreover, team members contribute to collective success through the concept of "team chemistry." Leaders must recognize the significance of team chemistry in selecting members and maximizing organizational outcomes. This multidimensional understanding serves as a foundation for developing strategies that nurture effective leadership and cohesive teamwork.
- Optimizing employee performance and well-being in individual and team settings demands a multifaceted approach that integrates stress-management interventions and embraces steadfast leadership. Stress management involves primary, secondary, and tertiary interventions. By addressing causal factors, reducing symptoms, and fostering rehabilitation, these interventions create a holistic framework for mitigating stress and trauma, which is particularly crucial in high-pressure environments such as healthcare.
- Steadfast leadership introduces a paradigm shift in decision-making by recognizing the importance of emotional intelligence (EQ) and nonrational faculties alongside traditional rationality. Leaders guided by intuition and emotional insights can enhance their understanding of employees. In the pursuit of organizational success, acknowledging and harnessing both rational and nonrational cognitive faculties can lead to a more resilient and thriving healthcare workforce.

Chapter 5

Measuring Outcomes to Improve Healthcare Success

The evolution of psychological principles has contributed to the widespread adoption of somatic psychology in myriads of healthcare settings. Despite their effectiveness, it remains difficult to assess their outcomes, especially when analyzing interventions that focus on the mind–body connection. This chapter aims to resolve this challenge by explaining how to identify feasible measures for assessing the outcomes of polyvagal-informed strategies. These clinical measures can be used by different parties with the underlying objective of improving how people perceive their emotional states following a specific intervention.

Objectives
- To understand the challenges of assessing the outcomes of somatic psychology interventions.
- To identify feasible measures for assessing the outcomes of polyvagal-informed strategies.
- To compare the strengths and outcomes of various clinical measures for assessing PVT outcomes.

> **Scenario: Why Can't I Prove Change?**
>
> As you may recall, one of the notable patients at Safe Haven is Fred Johnson, a 45-year-old man who is confronting the complexities of severe social anxiety. Fred often struggles to read social cues. His inability to understand people's expressions often pushes him to feel an exaggerated sense of threat. He feels like there is another person living inside him. When he is alone or with his family, he is usually calm and collected. However, as soon as he is exposed to a group setting he tends to sweat and feel on edge. This explains his tendency to avoid large social gatherings. He arrived at Safe Haven with the sole goal of overcoming his social anxiety, and he recognized that this may be a challenging and lengthy process.
>
> As soon as Fred arrives, Dr. Jennings's team recognizes his tendency to fluctuate up and down the polyvagal ladder. This behavior highlights his challenges in regulating his ANS responses. In response to Fred's social anxiety challenges, Dr. Jennings implements a holistic strategy rooted in the principles of the PVT. As a result, Fred becomes an active participant in his therapeutic journey by trying to understand the PVT, participating in mapping exercises, and delving into the intricacies of interoception and emotional regulation. Furthermore, both individual and group interventions have served as essential platforms for Fred's exploration of cues of safety. This recovery journey serves as an enlightening opportunity for Fred to strengthen the connection between his body and his mind.
>
> However, a major problem emerged four months into the process. As Fred traversed this therapeutic path, Dr. Jennings encountered difficulty in capturing the essence of his progress. The complexity of his condition, coupled with the intricacies of social anxiety, made

assessment a severe challenge. Dr. Jennings found herself in a scenario where the conventional measures of progress fell short.

Dr. Jennings deliberated whether to should use subjective measures to assess this patient's progress, but questioned whether they would provide her with an accurate assessment of Fred's well-being. If all else fails, she will observe his behavior in the long term and use objective measures to assess his physiological response. Her colleague has also recommended that she review several psychometric measures that can allow her to gain a glimpse of Fred's well-being. Considering the wide variety of clinical measures that currently exist, Dr. Jennings wonders how she should proceed in order to ascertain whether Fred Johnson is truly recovering from his social anxiety.

Challenges in Assessing PVT Intervention Outcomes

Assessing the outcomes of mental healthcare interventions has been a highly controversial issue for many years. One of the key challenges facing these measures lies in their focus on varying healthcare characteristics. The World Health Organization defines health as "a state of complete physical, mental, and social well-being, and not merely the absence of disease or infirmity" (www.who.int/about/governance/constitution). This definition highlights that good health consists of a person's recovery to normal functioning as well as the amelioration of undesirable symptoms and problems. However, the reality is that very few clinical measures focus on assessing a patient's development of protective factors, such as resilience, or the attainment of positive well-being.

The problem is worsened by the fact that most psychology interventions can only be assessed using subjective measures. Determining a patient's emotional or physiological response is a highly subjective process that can vary depending on the patient's inherent characteristics and/or the surrounding environmental factors. In some situations, there is a need to assess how a patient's well-being progresses over time. Such situations often emerge when subtle shifts in a person's behavior cannot conclusively determine the outcome of an intervention. Hence, the variability of many somatic psychology measures makes it incredibly challenging to arrive at accurate outcomes. Mental health interventions are also often broad because they tend to target individuals who are "struggling," experiencing moderate mental health issues, or "floundering" (Thomicroft and Slade 2014). Instead of viewing mental health as a state of being present or absent, it is better to perceive it as a continuum with varying levels.

At one end of the spectrum are individuals who are struggling with life difficulties, stressors, interpersonal issues, and other factors that affect their well-being. In the middle are individuals who are experiencing moderate mental health symptoms. Although these individuals are not in crisis or severe distress, there may be a substantial decline in the individual's day-to-day functioning. Finally, individuals who are floundering are often grappling with severe mental health issues, such as distress that compromises their overall well-being. That said, less than half of individuals who are struggling because of mental health issues are not detected in general practice settings because of the difficulty of identifying somatic symptoms (McFarlane et al. 2008). This spectrum of mental health can hinder a healthcare practitioner from making conclusive assessments about the state and well-being of a patient.

The evolving nature of mental health has contributed to the growing awareness that mental health has a broad spectrum and requires diverse interventions and support systems to improve patients' mental well-being. Furthermore, while traditional clinical measures focused on assessing the patient as the main target of study, it remains important to incorporate the well-being of other health stakeholders, such as healthcare staff; caregivers, such as family and friends; and members of the public (Thornicroft and Slad 2014). This can be achieved by using diverse clinical measures to assess outcomes.

Therefore, a good clinical measure should be multifaceted in terms of assessing the outcomes of polyvagal-informed strategies, and also conclusive in assessing intervention outcomes. Based on these challenges, today's healthcare professionals need to understand the benefits and drawbacks associated with different approaches to assessing polyvagal-informed interventions.

Measures for Assessing Mind–Body Outcomes

The regulation of emotional states is intricately linked to the physiological functions of the central nervous system (CNS), of which the ANS is a part. In simple words, the way people experience emotions is closely tied to the workings of the CNS. As a result, psychophysiological signals can provide valuable information about how emotional states influence brain activity. These signals offer insights into the dynamic interplay between the CNS and the peripheral nervous system (Moon et al. 2021). Additionally, they shed light on how the interaction between an individual's body and their surrounding environment can trigger psychophysiological responses. This leads back to the concept of neuroception and how external and internal stimuli can be seen as cues of danger or safety, thus triggering a shift along the polyvagal ladder to the corresponding state. This process is depicted in Figure 5.1.

Accordingly, analyzing various markers associated with the ANS can provide important information about how an individual responds to stress. The optimal or abnormal levels of

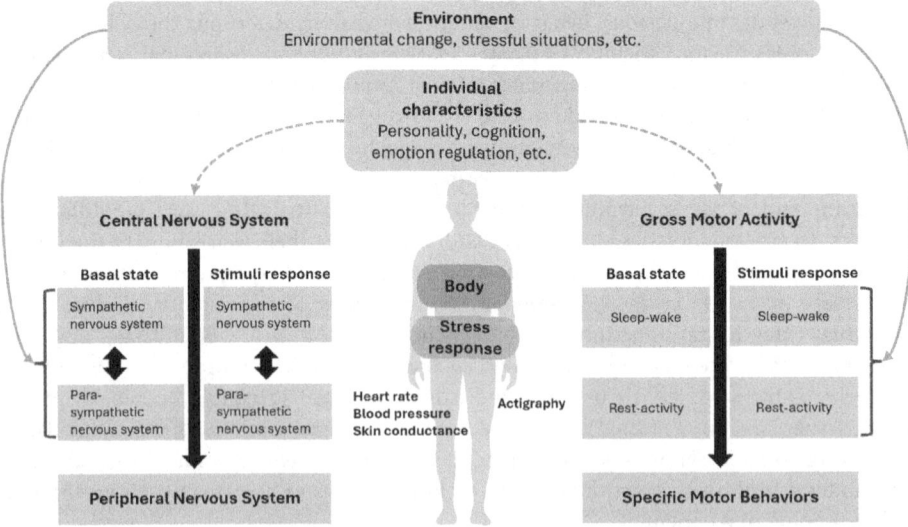

Figure 5.1 Measuring brain activity in response to environmental factors. External and internal stimuli can trigger a shift between sympathetic and PNS dominance, impacting motor behavior and physiological stress responses. (Source: Moon et al. 2021.)

these markers can give crucial insights into an individual's unique patterns when responding to stress, anxiety, or other emotional states. By measuring a person's physiological markers, such as heart rate, blood pressure, temperature, skin color, and pupil size, healthcare professionals can better understand how a person's body and mind react to and cope with stressors.

Feelings of safety are rooted in specific neurophysiological responses. Therefore, it is possible to measure the outcomes of related interventions using appropriate clinical measures. This rationale shifts the clinical measures from a realm primarily based on subjective experiences and perceptions to an objective and empirical scientific endeavor (Porges 2022, 1). By identifying the mental, physical, and emotional factors responsible for safety perceptions, researchers create a reliable framework for studying and enhancing an individual's sense of safety. These measures include objective measures, behavioral observations, subjective reports, and standardized psychological assessments, and can lead to the design and implementation of effective polyvagal-informed interventions.

Objective Measures

Objective measures are quantitative tools that provide a scientific foundation for assessing the impact of a certain intervention over a specific period of time. When evaluating longitudinal changes and predicting responses to therapeutic interventions, there are several key measures that serve as prominent phenotypic metrics. These metrics are instrumental in assessing how an individual's physiological responses and reactions may change over time and how they might respond to various forms of therapy. Among these metrics, some of the most clinically significant parameters when a person is at rest are heart rate (HR), heart-rate variability (HRV), respiratory sinus arrhythmia (RSA), and diastolic blood pressure (DBP) (Moon et al. 2021).

In comparison, there are several measures that can be used to clinically assess a person's reactivity to stressors. These include electrodermal activity (EDA), electromyography (EMG) startle response, eye movement and pupillometry, and facial EMG (Moon et al. 2021, 3). This tracking can help healthcare providers and patients observe trends and patterns, making it easier to identify when interventions are effective and whether adjustments are needed.

The most effective measures for polyvagal-informed interventions are provided in Table 5.1.

As with any measure, there are both benefits and drawbacks to using objective measures to assess PVT-focused outcomes. Objective measures often provide clear and quantifiable results, which is advantageous when evaluating specific aspects of the PVT. In addition, they are efficient and cost effective because they require minimal resources and can be applied without extensive training or equipment. Therefore, these instruments have a wide range of applications. However, objective measures often lead to rigid right-or-wrong thinking, which may not allow for the flexibility and adaptability required in understanding complex phenomena. Objective measures simply may not capture the holistic picture of the PVT. Remember, this is a comprehensive theory that involves physiological, psychological, and social components. Therefore, objective measures may excel in assessing certain physiological aspects (e.g., HR variability), but they can fall short in evaluating the psychological and social dimensions.

Table 5.1 Objective measures for polyvagal-informed interventions

At Rest	Reacting to Stressors
Heart Rate (HR): A lower resting heart rate is often associated with a well-functioning PNS, promoting relaxation and social engagement.	**Electrodermal Activity (EDA):** EDA, or skin conductance, can reveal emotional arousal or a shift toward sympathetic activation in response to an impending threat.
Heart-Rate Variability (HRV): A higher HRV typically signifies a more adaptive ANS, highlighting a person's ability to respond flexibly to environmental challenges and recover from stressors.	**Electromyography (EMG) Startle Response:** The startle response, as measured by EMG, is indicative of the body's quick, defensive reactions when preparing the body for a fight-or-flight response.
Respiratory Sinus Arrhythmia (RSA): Greater RSA suggests that an individual's vagus nerve is effectively modulating HR in response to breathing, indicating readiness for social engagement and relaxation.	**Eye Movement and Pupillometry:** The movement of the eyes and changes in pupil size reflect how individuals visually engage with the environment and respond emotionally to social cues.
Diastolic Blood Pressure (DBP): A well-regulated parasympathetic system may lead to lower diastolic blood pressure during rest, indicating a more relaxed state.	**Facial EMG:** Recording electrical activity in facial muscles can provide insights into the connection between facial expressions and the capacity for social engagement and emotional regulation.

A balanced approach that combines objective measures with other methods, such as self-report questionnaires and qualitative assessments, can provide a more comprehensive understanding of the PVT's impact on individuals' well-being and social interactions.

> **Case Study 5.1: Tracking Fred's Physiology**
>
> Dr. Jennings has considered several clinical measures that can allow her to understand Fred's physiological responses and reactions following the interventions. Objective measures can provide reliable evidence regarding his improvement. Among them, the simplest ones involve monitoring Fred's HR variability and DBP. In addition, an eye movement and pupillometry test can assess how he visually engages with his environment.
>
> Dr. Jennings establishes a baseline by assessing Fred's responses when he is alone and when he is in a group setting. These objective measures offer her clear and quantifiable results regarding his problem, and they are quite cost effective. However, Dr. Jennings feels that these measures are too rigid because they cannot offer her a coherent picture of the outcomes of her team's interventions.
>
> Perhaps objective measures are not adequate for determining whether Fred's social anxiety problems are resolving.

Subjective Reports

While objective measures and behavioral reports usually require concrete data for one to draw accurate conclusions, subjective reports are usually dependent on direct feedback from the patients (Miller and Lovler 2018). These instruments can shed light on the patient's mental and emotional state by assessing their opinions, insights, and experiences. The patients may provide information regarding their stress levels, anxiety levels, and feelings of safety. A suitable metric for assessing the efficacy of polyvagal-informed interventions is emotional well-being (EWB), which is linked to physical health, healthy aging, and longevity. Over the years, there has been a proliferation of theories, constructs, and measures related to emotional well-being, leading to a diverse shift in EWB research across healthcare and other disciplines. Subjective reports that assess EWB can allow healthcare practitioners to understand the patient's internal world.

Subjective reports have significant benefits, as well as drawbacks. On the one hand, they excel in capturing the patient's emotions, thoughts, experiences, and perceptions. Considering that the PVT emphasizes the importance of understanding an individual's physiological and emotional responses, subjective reports can offer valuable insights into how a person subjectively experiences stress, safety, and social engagement. Furthermore, an individual can describe their experiences as they encounter them.

On the other hand, a key limitation of subjective reports is the lack of consistent metrics for assessing psychological outcomes. For example, it can be exceedingly challenging to assess EWB because its definitions vary widely based on a practitioner's training, areas of interest, and the target populations (Koslouski et al. 2022). This diversity of definitions and measures poses challenges in the communication and dissemination of research findings. In addition, subjective reports are highly susceptible to biases because patients may fail to report their experiences truthfully, or they may experience difficulty articulating their feelings and perceptions. These limitations need to be addressed before a healthcare practitioner uses such reports to evaluate the outcomes of polyvagal-informed interventions.

> **Case Study 5.2: Subjective Reporting**
>
> Using subjective reports was another one of Dr. Jennings's initial ideas for assessing Fred's progress. Subjective reports are particularly suitable for capturing the patient's emotions, thoughts, and experiences after undergoing the interventions. These reports focus on his stress levels, anxiety levels, feelings of safety, and EWB. Subjective reports can capture the interplay between his physiological and emotional states and allow him to describe his experiences using his own words.
>
> Nonetheless, Dr. Jennings is still concerned that the subjective reports are not an adequate approach for concluding Fred's case. While Dr. Jennings doesn't necessarily think it's likely, Fred could lie about his outcomes or, at the very least, his opinions may be influenced by prejudice or other factors.
>
> The low accuracy of subjective reports encourages Dr. Jennings to consider alternatives for assessing Fred Johnson's outcomes.

Behavioral Observation

Compared to objective measures, behavioral observations offer real-world evidence of how successfully patients are applying polyvagal-informed strategies to their daily lives. These tests primarily focus on monitoring a person's behavior and how the individual responds in a given context (Miller and Lovler 2018). As a result, they can reveal whether the skills nurtured through the polyvagal-informed interventions translate into positive improvements in the patient's behaviors. These observations usually focus on various dimensions of the patients' lives, such as social engagement and emotional regulation. The observations ensure that healthcare professionals consider the full spectrum of the patient's health and well-being.

Behavioral observations can serve as a critical bridge between theory and practice in the context of the PVT. By analyzing how patients apply polyvagal-informed strategies in real-world situations, clinicians can assess the effectiveness of these interventions and tailor their therapeutic approaches to meet their client's mental health needs. Behavioral observation allows for a more holistic evaluation of the patient's progress by providing a mechanism for refining and optimizing the application of the PVT in clinical settings. This integration of theory into observable, real-life outcomes is vital for delivering comprehensive and patient-centered care.

However, despite their effectiveness, healthcare professionals should also recognize the limitations of behavioral observation. Foremost, reactivity and observer effect are common problems. When individuals being observed are aware of the presence of observers, reactivity can occur (Kamphaus and Tsushima 2016). In the context of the PVT, this means that individuals may change their behavior because they know they are being watched.

This limitation is particularly relevant when assessing how individuals naturally apply polyvagal-informed strategies in real-life situations. Events that trigger these behaviors may not be common and may be difficult to replicate in an artificial observational evaluation. These low-frequency behaviors can be challenging to capture through behavioral observation, which can hinder the healthcare professional from discerning polyvagal-related responses. Moreover, behavioral observation can be labor intensive, time consuming, and costly. Significant personnel and logistical costs can be a barrier, especially when extensive observations are needed.

> **Case Study 5.3: Observing Fred**
>
> Fred Johnson has been a long-time patient at Safe Haven Clinic, so behavioral observation is a possible approach for assessing his progress in overcoming social anxiety. For that reason, Dr. Jennings assigns one of her subordinates to assess Fred's behavior during social interactions. The observer will focus on his body language, eye contact, and overall engagement. The results of the observation will provide Dr. Jennings with tangible evidence of the outcomes of the polyvagal-informed interventions in real-life situations.
>
> Nonetheless, the main problem is that Fred may alter his behavior when he realizes he is being observed, and unconsented observation may raise ethical concerns. Furthermore, the process is quite costly because it requires Dr. Jennings to allocate a worker to monitor Fred. These problems convince her that behavioral observation is a poor long-term solution for assessing this patient's progress.

Standardized Psychological Assessments

Standardized psychological assessments can also be utilized to measure specific psychological constructs. Briefly defined, a *psychological construct* is a label applied to a set of behaviors that are seen to be grouped together commonly under certain conditions. For example, if someone is seen as nervously biting their nails, trembling, and looking around furtively, one could infer that they are anxious about some situation.

Measurement of constructs relies on the use of instruments that are explicitly designed to measure response to the studied intervention or to multiple interventions (Miller and Lovler 2018). These assessments provide structured measures, allowing healthcare professionals to track changes in patients' mental and EWB over time. The most reliable measures include stress scales, depression scales, anxiety scales, body awareness and perception measures, safety and social engagement measures, sensory processing measures, and well-being and life satisfaction measures.

Standardized psychometric measures have significant strengths and weaknesses. The most noticeable strength lies in the ability to provide clear and quantifiable information regarding a specific psychological construct. In addition, these tests are based on years of trials and experiments, so they are extremely reliable compared to other clinical measures. Furthermore, standardized psychological tests are less susceptible to bias because they are usually developed through a rigorous process with the objective of acquiring valid and reliable results. These benefits explain why many healthcare professionals rely on standardized psychometric measures to assess mental health outcomes.

However, it is also crucial to recognize the weaknesses of such measures. For instance, these instruments often lack depth because they cannot capture complex social, emotional, or behavioral responses. In addition to low flexibility, the instruments' overemphasis on quantification may encourage professionals to oversimplify psychological phenomena when more comprehensive assessments should be conducted. Overall, standardized psychological measures have gained popularity due to their accuracy, but their main weakness lies in their low flexibility.

Somatic and Psychological Health Scales

Somatic and psychological health scales are instruments designed to assess a wide combination of somatic and psychological responses. These scales are relatively unique because they can provide critical information about the physical and mental dimensions of a patient's recovery, whereas conventional psychology scales focus on the mental health dimensions. For instance, the Somatic and Psychological Health Report (SPHERE) is a 34-item questionnaire that can be administered in primary care and general care settings. Due to the large number of patients who do not receive care because they do not display significant somatic symptoms, SPHERE is designed to identify various indicators of psychological or somatic distress.

Stress Scales

Given that stress, depression, and anxiety are major triggers that can cause a person's autonomic state to shift in an undesirable way, it is essential to use measures that can analyze their severity within a patient. These measures can provide valuable insights to healthcare professionals about stress-related symptoms and issues. A suitable example is the Posttraumatic Stress Disorder (PTSD) Scale. This scale is a 17-item self-reported questionnaire that encourages respondents to provide crucial details regarding their traumatic experiences.

Depression Scales

Depression scales typically include questions that assess the frequency and severity of depressive symptoms. They usually provide a quantitative score that indicates the level of depression, with higher scores indicating more severe symptoms. For example, Patient

Health Questionnaire-9 (PHQ-9) is an evidence-based scale for assessing depression. This scale is a multipurpose instrument that can screen, diagnose, monitor, and measure a patient's severity of depression.

Anxiety Scales

Similar to depression scales, anxiety scales provide an objective and standardized assessment of anxiety levels. Such scales are quite reliable for monitoring changes in anxiety symptoms during and after the implementation of the polyvagal-informed intervention. In this context, Generalized Anxiety Disorder-7 (GAD-7) is one of the most reliable scales for assessing anxiety levels in a patient. This scale is a self-reported questionnaire often used to screen and measure the severity of anxiety disorder.

Body Awareness and Perception Measures

Body awareness and perception measures assess an individual's awareness of internal bodily sensations and their emotional significance, as developed by Stephen Porges and available through his nonprofit organization, the Polyvagal Institute. These measures are highly relevant to the PVT because they align with the theory's emphasis on interoception – the awareness of internal bodily states. The PVT highlights the importance of recognizing and interpreting bodily sensations as they relate to emotional states and ANS responses.

Safety and Social Engagement Measures

The Neuroception of Psychological Safety Scale assesses an individual's perception of safety in social interactions and is available through the Polyvagal Institute. This measure is directly aligned with the PVT, which emphasizes the importance of feeling safe and socially connected as a means of promoting an individual's overall well-being. The PVT posits that a sense of safety is a fundamental requirement for accessing the social engagement system and regulating the ANS. Therefore, assessments such as the Neuroception of Psychological Safety Scale help evaluate the effectiveness of interventions in creating a safe environment conducive to social engagement, which is a core aspect of the PVT.

Sensory Processing Measures

The Brain-Body Center Sensory Scale evaluates sensory processing and sensitivity. Sensory processing measures can allow a practitioner to understand how different individuals respond to their environments and how sensory input can trigger ANS responses. The PVT suggests that interventions should focus on regulating sensory input to support emotional regulation and well-being. That said, sensory processing measures can be employed to determine whether a patient has atypical responses to sensory input.

Well-Being and Life Satisfaction Measures

Well-being and life satisfaction are central concerns in the PVT. The Purpose in Life Scale measures an individual's sense of purpose and meaning in life, which are interconnected with overall well-being. The PVT recognizes that social engagement and the experience of safety are essential for enhancing one's quality of life. Assessments such as the Purpose in Life Scale help clinicians and researchers determine the impact of polyvagal-informed interventions on an individual's sense of purpose and life satisfaction. The Purpose in Life Scale is a 12-item instrument that assesses a patient's drive and sense of purpose in life.

Case Study 5.4: Measuring Fred's Anxiety

After reviewing objective measures, subjective measures, and behavioral observation, Dr. Jennings has decided to employ standardized psychometric measures. Various measures exist that focus on specific aspects of Fred's social anxiety. These measures include the SPHERE questionnaire, which can allow her to understand Fred's somatic and psychological responses. In comparison, stress scales such as the PTSD Scale can explain his stress levels, while depression scales such as the PHQ-9 are specifically designed to describe his depression levels. Alternatively, the anxiety scale (GAD-7) can provide crucial information regarding Fred's social anxiety, which is the root cause of his dysregulation.

In addition to these measures, there are several measures designed to focus on Fred's body awareness and perception, as well as his safety and social engagement. While the first category of instruments targets his internal body sensations, the second category focuses on his ability to identify cues of safety in his surroundings. With knowledge of these measures, Dr. Jennings has a general idea about the direction of her future assessments.

Key Takeaways

- Although there's been significant progress in mental health assessments, the field of somatic psychology still has room for further development. Foremost, mental health interventions focus on a broad spectrum of somatic and psychological issues, so healthcare professionals may fail to identify individuals who are in severe distress. Furthermore, mental health is also evolving because of the growing demand for services in our increasingly stress-filled world. Nowadays, mental health interventions consider healthcare staff, the patients' caregivers, and members of the public. For that reason, clinical measures should also recognize the importance of these stakeholders by ensuring their overall well-being following an intervention.
- Over the years, several clinical measures have been designed that focus on specific dimensions of the mind and the body. For instance, objective measures are inherently suitable for assessing physiological changes by assessing changes in HR, breathing, eye movement, and facial expressions. Although information acquired from these tests is usually reliable, a healthcare provider may struggle to understand the relations between different variables. Healthcare providers can also use subjective measures, but these instruments usually rely on information provided by the patient. Alternatively, behavioral observation is one of the oldest approaches for assessing PVT outcomes, but this approach carries significant expenses and labor requirements. The final strategy is to employ standardized psychological assessments. These tests often demonstrate outstanding results when assessing specific variables, but they are quite rigid compared to the other measures.
- There is no one-size-fits-all approach to mental health measures. Each measure has unique advantages and disadvantages, which makes it appropriate for certain situations and inappropriate in others. Thus, a multifaceted approach can play the greatest role in improving the assessment of polyvagal-informed interventions. Objective assessments can be utilized to acquire a baseline of the patient's responses before and after undergoing the polyvagal-informed interventions. Afterward, subjective reports can be utilized to understand the patient's experiences throughout

the interventions. Behavioral observation (under consent) can also be employed to monitor behavioral changes during the interventions. Finally, a standardized psychological test can be administered to determine whether the patient's well-being improved after participating in the interventions. This sequence offers a more reliable approach for determining a patient's progress than utilizing a single clinical measure.

Chapter 6
Designing Healthcare Environments That Promote Well-Being

Appealing building designs and workplace layouts can emphasize cues of safety while reducing cues of threat. With the evolution of healthcare concepts highlighting not just physical health but also mental and emotional health, the healthcare industry has begun to acknowledge the rising importance of conducive and appealing workplace designs and settings. While healthcare facilities serve crucial functions for sustaining key necessities, they are also essential for creating a sense of safety among the staff, patients, visitors, and other stakeholders. This chapter highlights the importance of various building elements, such as open floorplans, natural spaces, private areas, emergency-preparedness structures, inclusive designs, and appealing scents and sounds. Visually appealing and easy-to-navigate layouts can make a drastic difference in a facility's performance by promoting social engagement and strengthening the sense of safety.

Objectives
- To explain the influence of environmental factors on a person's perceptions of safety.
- To identify the building elements that strengthen the sense of safety for healthcare professionals.
- To describe the impact of conducive workplace layouts on healthcare workers' sense of safety.

Scenario: A Blueprint for Revitalizing Safe Haven

Dr. Reginald White is the CEO of Safe Haven Medical Clinic. The facility serves as a beacon of healthcare delivery in the region, making it a popular social amenity. However, the facility has become relatively outdated since its establishment in the early 1970s. As the CEO, Dr. White is responsible for assessing the need for structural changes.

Although attempts have been made to renovate and modernize the infrastructure, the facility has not succeeded in improving accessibility and safety for the occupants and visitors. There are no open spaces, and there is poor natural lighting in most rooms. In addition, the building was designed with efficiency as the sole goal, so there are few private spaces. Although emergency-preparedness structures are available, as evidenced by the number of ramps, elevators, and fire assembly points in the facility, there are certain concerns that have not been properly addressed, such as the inadequacy of emergency exits. Dr. White has been advised by an inspector that, at the moment, the building is still structurally sound. He knows he needs to promote safety within the walls but doesn't know how.

In the past, the facility underwent a series of renovations aimed at improving the aesthetic appeal, but the clinic continues to record low employee satisfaction owing to a poor work environment. Some workers have been complaining about suffocating room layouts, monotonous wall colors, poor navigation paths, and the lack of decor. These problems are worsened by the high noise levels and poor ventilation in most wards and offices.

Although these issues do not directly affect healthcare delivery, they do influence the workers' mood and overall productivity. Dr. White is overwhelmed by the list of issues mentioned by the workers. While some issues can be easily resolved, financial limitations may hinder him from addressing all issues. He needs to consider feasible solutions for making alterations that convey safety to workers, patients, and other visitors to the clinic.

The Impact of Environmental Factors on the Sense of Safety

As you now know, the PVT emphasizes the need to understand the internal sensations that contribute to engagement (ventral vagal state), mobilization (sympathetic state), or immobilization/disengagement (the dorsal vagal state). However, it is also essential to remember that the surrounding environment tends to have a profound impact on the process of neuroception – that is, whether the ANS perceives danger or safety (see Chapter 1: "Interoception and Neuroception").

The ANS is highly attuned to subtle changes in the environment. The passive pathways that promote social engagement usually rely on the senses to send appropriate signals of danger or safety. This explains why a building positioned in a neighborhood with poor architecture, no greenery, poor accessibility, and neglected maintenance is likely to make inhabitants feel unsafe. In comparison, neighborhoods with wide walking paths and better environmental quality often provide higher levels of perceived safety (Zeng et al. 2022). These findings underscore the significance of creating conducive healthcare environments that stimulate social engagement.

Due to neuroception and interoception, most people have an innate awareness of the influence of their environment on their safety. Subtle environmental cues involving lighting, acoustics, and ambiance can strengthen the sense of safety and, in turn, encourage social engagement. Positive sensory comfort tends to activate the socialization state and hinder shifts toward mobilization and immobilization. In the healthcare environment, which is often characterized by high stress and trauma, it is integral to alter the work environment to promote health and well-being.

Temperature and Ventilation

Considerable research has been published pertaining to the link between the surrounding thermal environment and the inhabitants' physiological and mental well-being. "Thermal discomfort" is a term associated with extreme thermal environments (Ahmed et al. 2022). Changes in the internal temperature trigger a conditional stimulus that influences the skin and other key organs to return the body to its optimal temperature levels. In such situations, thermal discomfort can easily lead to a decline in a worker's productivity and overall behavior. In this context, extremely high or low temperatures can sway the ANS to be attentive to cues of danger because the body perceives the elements as external threats. Therefore, thermal comfort has become a crucial consideration in creating a conducive work environment.

Given that the majority of healthcare workers spend most of their time indoors, healthcare facilities must ensure that they are providing good airflow and temperature conditions to instill a sense of safety in the occupants and optimize employee productivity.

Cooling, heating, and ventilation are the most reliable strategies for mitigating thermal discomfort in the workplace. This goal can be achieved through artificial strategies, such as the installation of cooling devices and ventilation machines to control airflow, temperature, and humidity. The presence of open spaces and sightlines for airflow also contribute to mitigating thermal discomfort.

> **Case Study 6.1: Improving the Environment**
>
> Among the challenges noted at Safe Haven Medical Clinic, poor ventilation and thermal discomfort were identified by the staff as critical issues. The facility was often too hot and stuffy in some areas and too cool in others. These high and low temperatures often led to physical discomfort in the staff, thereby triggering the flight-or-fight response. Some complained of fatigue because their work areas were too warm, and others found themselves chilled from the vents directly above their workstations.
>
> Dr. White has already recommended the removal of a few walls for a more open-plan layout, and he knows that this will improve airflow. However, he wants to create a work environment that is characterized by optimal humidity and temperature conditions. He suggests that the facility undergo a revamp of the heating and air-conditioning system with a long-term maintenance plan. Placement of the office furniture and equipment will need to be carefully considered when the new layout is configured so that no employee is directly under the vents.

The Importance of Appealing Design

Human structures were initially designed with the primary objective of protecting the inhabitants from the elements. As humanity progressed, the focus gradually shifted from safety and security to comfort and aesthetics. Accordingly, a designer must consider various features, such as accessibility, traffic, needs, and emergency mitigation. For instance, the vast majority of mental health institutions are designed with calming neutral colors to create a soothing atmosphere for the clients.

Instead of the traditional work environment, wherein workers are isolated as they strive to complete their daily quotas, the science of safety recommends a more conducive environment that stimulates the VVC to maintain the social engagement system. The main goal then is to create a workplace setting where employees are inclined to socialize with one another while delivering to their full potential. In short, the physical environment of an office, reception area, or building can affect a person's physiology by encouraging them to make rapid judgments about whether the location is safe based on the evident cues of safety. By carefully tailoring the location, it is possible to convey a story to the visitors that subconsciously informs them that they are welcome (Dana 2018).

Simple factors such as a building's size, shape, material texture, color, balance, symmetry, space, pattern, and decoration can influence the viewer's perceptions. Aesthetically pleasing buildings are not only appealing to the inhabitants, they can also enhance their surroundings. For instance, studies reveal that access to natural light can improve students' academic outcomes, and well-lit environments can reduce workers' stress levels and strengthen their job satisfaction levels (Awada et al. 2023).

Similarly, designing spaces that are open and have good visibility can encourage the occupants to feel safer in their surroundings. Large windows, skylights, and lightwells can transform a facility by strengthening its connection to nature. By reducing blind spots and potential hiding spots, designers can create open spaces with clear visibility. The developer can position structures to optimize natural lighting inside and outside the structure. Within these well-lit and open spaces, it is easier to monitor the surroundings, which can foster openness and safety among the workers. Although natural lighting is preferable, developers can enhance the sense of safety of a building using artificial light. The natural interplay between nature and manmade structures can bring a unique character to a healthcare facility that is perceived as welcoming.

In addition, incorporating nature in the building design can create a soothing ambiance for the occupants. Research reveals that natural sunlight can positively strengthen the regulation of one's circadian rhythm and allow the occupants to sleep better (Blume et al. 2019). This, in turn, results in improved health. Nature is often associated with a calming and stress-reducing impact on the senses, thereby creating an imaginary sense of connection to the environment. Nature can be incorporated into a building's design through various strategies. For instance, the developer can introduce plants, water features (including fishponds or aquariums), and other natural aspects to create a calming environment. Embracing nature is a sustainable architectural strategy that is beneficial to the building's environment and to the immediate stakeholders by promoting a sense of calm and well-being.

Designers can also incorporate private spaces that strengthen the sense of personal comfort and safety in patients, healthcare workers, and visitors. Visitors may enjoy a comfortable waiting area where they can wait at ease, while the workers may benefit from a staff lounge with access to food and beverages. Workers can take breaks in these rooms and recharge after dealing with heavy workloads. In addition, these comfortable spaces can also serve as the location for staff meetings, serving as collaborative workspaces for promoting teamwork and communication.

Another critical consideration in building design is emergency preparedness. Healthcare facilities are unique compared to conventional buildings because they usually require multiple exits to facilitate the entry and exit of patients during high patient influx. Furthermore, the existence of public spaces where everyone can gather during emergencies communicates safety. In these areas, individuals can easily identify the best route to reach safety in emergencies. The knowledge that there is a direct path to safety can encourage the occupants to relax. Other emergency-preparedness features include shelter areas, training and drill spaces, and emergency exits.

Finally, designers should also consider social and cultural diversity. For instance, an important social factor is disability. People with physical disabilities usually require accessible avenues for movement, such as ramps, elevators, and escalators. These structures are essential for meeting the needs of marginalized groups who struggle with social disability.

Another important cultural factor is local heritage. Healthcare facilities positioned in diverse or Indigenous areas often incorporate the local community by creating healthcare structures that complement their culture. A facility based on culturally reflective architectural designs can demonstrate respect for the local aesthetics of its patients and the wider community.

Case Study 6.2: Promoting Cues of Safety in Design

Dr. White needs to implement several recommendations to ensure the clinic is perceived as safe by workers, patients, and other individuals. For instance, he recommends the redesign of certain areas to improve lighting by creating spaces for large windows, skylights, sightlines, and open spaces. In addition, he designates specific sections of the clinic to serve as waiting areas or staff lounges. These areas can serve multiple purposes, including providing comfort and facilitating social interactions.

Another suitable recommendation is to create avenues and channels for emergency exits. By conducting a comprehensive evaluation of emergency preparedness, Dr. White can identify critical deficiencies that may induce a sense of danger in the workplace. Furthermore, the interior design can also be altered to match the social and cultural values of the key stakeholders. These recommendations necessitate Safe Haven Clinic to allocate significant funds for structural redevelopment. Despite the financial costs of the recommendations, the proposed changes can positively influence the perceptions of workers, patients, and other stakeholders for years to come.

The Importance of Conducive Workplace Layouts

While it is not always possible to alter the external environment, it is feasible to alter a healthcare facility's interior to promote safety. Considering that most workers spend many hours in their workplace, a conveniently designed building can inspire and encourage them to work to their full potential. Simple features – such as sound, temperature, and scent – can influence the workers' polyvagal state, leaning them toward the ventral vagal state when thoughtfully provided.

The field of environmental psychology has attempted to investigate the immediate influence of working environment on employees at the individual and organizational levels (Kwon and Remøy 2020). In recent years, researchers have noted a stronger association between office comfort and employee satisfaction. These findings emerge from the idea that lack of privacy and territorialism is a significant obstacle to employee satisfaction and productivity. Other factors that need to be considered to create conducive workplace layouts are visual appeal, aroma, sound, temperature, and ventilation. By creating optimal workplace layouts, healthcare facilities can improve their employees' response to stressors and their perception of safety.

Visual Appeal

Visual appeal tends to have a positive impact on workers' mental health and EWB. A study conducted at the University of Michigan highlighted the importance of visual appeal and color in cognition (Kaplan, Kaplan, and Ryan 1998). According to the researchers, the primary objective was to investigate how humans react to their visual environments. The findings reveal that human beings often seek familiar objects or constructs when they are placed in new environments; this allows them to determine whether the surrounding is welcoming or intimidating. That said, lighting serves a crucial role by highlighting building elements, spaces, and textures in a manner that creates feelings of familiarity.

A comprehensive evaluation of the factors that contribute to a building's visual appeal is necessary to explain how they can provide cues of safety to individuals.

- **Lighting.** With regard to lighting, the most important factors are brightness, hue, and saturation. Brightness describes the amount of light produced by a light source, and it is known to affect a person's emotions. For example, bright lights can intensify a person's emotions, whereas low light can keep them steady or reduce their emotional affect. Hue is known to affect a person's happiness. For instance, studies show that natural light

Table 6.1 The psychological impact of different lighting effects

Psychological Impact	Lighting Effect	Light Distribution
Tense	Intense direct light from above	Nonuniform
Relaxed	Lower overhead lighting with some lighting at room perimeter, warm tones	Nonuniform
Work/Visual Clarity	Bright light on work plane with less light at the perimeter, wall lighting, cooler tones	Uniform
Spaciousness	Bright light with lighting on walls and possibly ceiling	Uniform
Privacy/Intimacy	Low light level at activity space with a little perimeter lighting and dark areas in rest of space	Nonuniform

Source: TCP Lighting (2017).

tends to make people happier than artificial light, so organizations should seek a convenient balance of artificial and natural lighting to improve their buildings' visual appeal. Saturation defines the intensity of a color. Similar to brightness, highly saturated hues can amplify a person's emotions, whereas low saturation tends to dampen the target's emotions. These three elements can be altered to evoke a specific psychological impact on workers, as illustrated in Table 6.1.

- **Layout.** The office layout can determine whether employees feel safe in their respective surroundings. For instance, when looking at open-ended and close-ended office layouts, occupants can easily identify significant differences. Cubicle-based layouts are usually arranged to ensure the optimal use of office space, rather than prioritizing the employees' needs. As a result, a close-ended layout can create a "suffocating" sensation. In contrast, open-ended workplace layouts are more convenient for collaboration and social engagement than close-ended layouts. These workplaces are often characterized by a higher degree of visibility and stronger communication among the workers than close-ended layouts. Thus, the visual appeal of the workplace layout can dictate the depth of social interactions between the workers.
- **Color.** In addition to open spaces, vibrant work environments can also strengthen the sense of safety of a facility's inhabitants. A vibrant workplace refers to a lively and energetic layout that creates an uplifting atmosphere. Color can be a powerful psychological tool for altering a person's mood and attitude. Color therapy, or chromotherapy, is a technique that uses color to balance the body's energy centers (based on the concept of chakras, rooted in ancient Hinduism and Buddhism) and to treat specific physical and mental health conditions (Jogdand 2022). This therapy is derived from the idea that warm colors, such as red, orange, and yellow, are often associated with positive work environments and emotional states. In some cases, they can stimulate people and make them more excited. Some individuals believe that each color has a specific meaning and can evoke a specific psychological response in a person. One could argue that excitatory colors are more likely to activate a shift to sympathetic or ventral vagal states, whereas soothing, calming colors would tend to shift the nervous

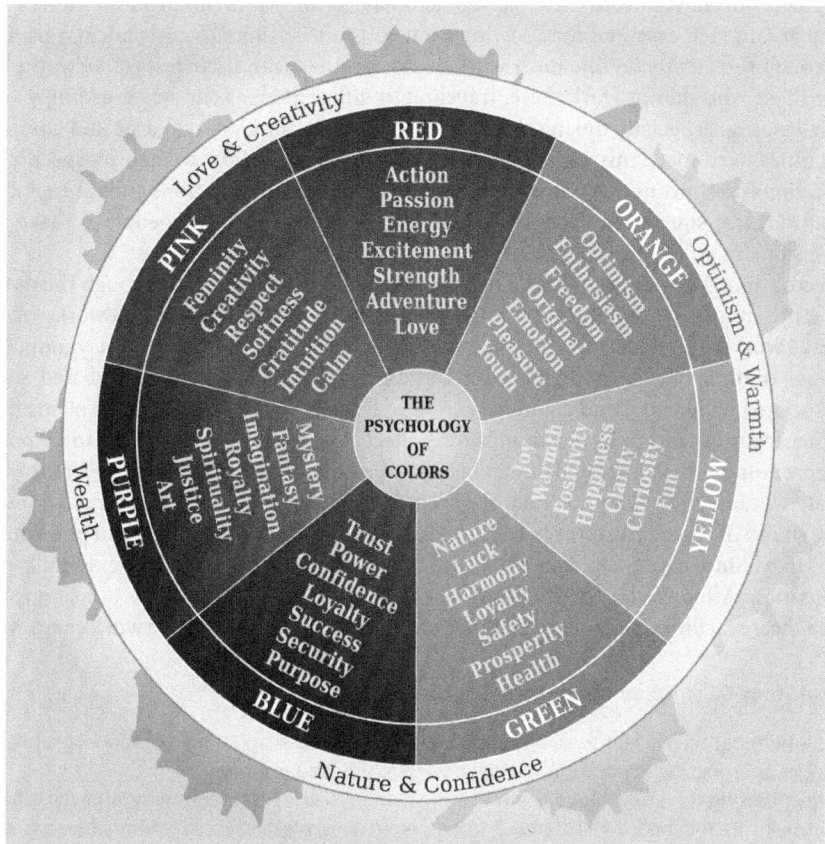

Figure 6.1 Color psychology wheel. (Source: Authors)

system from a sympathetic to a calmer ventral vagal state. Use of color has not been associated with trying to induce a dorsal vagal state; however, we could see how warm and gently activating colors might help shift a person out of immobilization. For example, many individuals associate blue with positive calming influences. A color psychology chart, such as the one shown in Figure 6.1, can be used to select colors that may evoke particular nervous system states on the polyvagal ladder.
- Using the color psychology wheel, it is possible to design the workplace to optimize productivity using one or more colors. For instance, a combination of blue, green, and yellow could convey feelings of confidence, safety, harmony, warmth, and positivity to influence patients in a positive way. These colors are significant in the healthcare sector because of their ability to encourage states of relaxation, safety, warmth, and even joy. If we consider how a particular color may be activating or calming, we can map this to which polyvagal ladder state may be promoted by the use of single or combined colors. A suitable workplace setting would involve soothing colors, look clean, and provide ample bright (but not harsh) lighting.

- **Signage and navigation.** Clear signage and navigation paths can promote cues of safety and are, in fact, essential for allowing occupants and visitors to conveniently navigate through the facility. While most workers are familiar with their respective workplaces, for those who do not work there, traveling to different areas can be exceedingly challenging, especially during times of stress, trauma, or anxiety. Large and complex facilities need mechanisms for communicating to visitors how to identify specific locations on short notice. These areas include fire assembly locations and emergency exit routes. Clear signage can alleviate stress and confusion, allowing people to make quick decisions in an unfamiliar environment.
- **Decoration.** The aesthetic appeal of a facility can also be improved through the use of creative interiors and decoration. A thoughtfully and carefully decorated workspace can make workers feel safe and eliminate adverse emotional influences that may induce fear, stress, trauma, or anxiety. In addition, certain types of decor are evidence-based and associated with a cool and calming sensation. For example, Dana (2018) explains that water features tend to have a diminishing effect on a person's stress levels and a positive impact on their well-being. Human beings usually have an evolutionary reverence for water because of its unique restorative properties. Accordingly, looking at water or hearing the sound of waves, rivers, or brooks can restore a person's psyche and send powerful cues of safety. Similarly, green decorations involving exotic plants can achieve a similar sensation. Although creative interiors and decoration do not serve a functional purpose in healthcare facilities, they are integral for creating a safe and conducive work environment.

> **Case Study 6.3: Improving the Visual Appeal**
>
> Dr. White identified clear weaknesses in the facility's visual appeal that induce a sense of danger and uncertainty among the clinic's occupants and visitors.
>
> Recognizing the importance of visual appeal on EWB, the first recommendation Dr. White will make to the board is to create open-ended workplace layouts where the staff can collaborate and engage with one another when not dealing directly with patients. This involves removing a few walls in some key areas and reorganizing the placement of the workstations.
>
> His second recommendation is to repaint the entire facility, choosing a blend of vibrant colors that communicate Safe Haven's mission and vision. For instance, he will specifically suggest white, blue, and orange as these have been identified as colors that communicate openness, organization, and good energy.
>
> His third recommendation is for improved signage and navigation paths to reduce stress and confusion among patients and visitors; his fourth and final recommendation involves redecorating the facility with a focus on evidence-based approaches. For instance, water features are often associated with a calming and stress-reducing work environment, so he'll suggest installing a wall fountain between the patient waiting area and the main work area.
>
> These approaches are relatively more affordable than a complete redesign of the building.

Key Takeaways

- Numerous environmental factors can influence a person's perception of safety. According to the PVT, the ANS is highly attuned to assess cues of safety and danger by examining the surroundings.

- Research reveals that factors such as architecture, lighting, and accessibility can heighten a person's awareness of their perceived safety. Therefore, it is possible to alter the environmental factors to trigger positive sensory stimuli in patients, healthcare workers, and other stakeholders.
- Good ventilation and consistent cooling/heating reduces thermal discomfort, thereby improving employee satisfaction and productivity.
- Appealing building designs serve a more important purpose than improving the aesthetic appeal. Nowadays, developers of healthcare buildings need to assess how the physical environment and the size, shape, texture, color, balance, symmetry, decor, and space of structures affect the viewer's perception of safety.
- To improve cues of safety, research recommends the following: incorporating natural and artificial light where appropriate, designing open and visible spaces for easier sightlines, integrating nature in building designs, creating private spaces for patients and healthcare workers, ensuring emergency preparedness, and considering social and cultural diversity when designing a healthcare facility.

Chapter 7
Interfacing with External Stakeholders

No exploration of developing and running a healthcare organization is complete without some focus on relationships with external stakeholders, which are broadly defined as payors, regulators, community leaders and members, and ancillary support staff (such as first responders). This chapter shifts the focus toward key external stakeholders involved in the funding and support of healthcare facilities. These stakeholders include payors, healthcare providers, learning institutions, and community-based organizations.

It is worth exploring if there are ways to incorporate the PVT into interactions with these stakeholders and how that might help with clinical and financial outcomes. In addition, it is useful to examine the strategies for marketing such programs and presenting their outcomes to the public. This chapter marks the final step in implementing polyvagal-informed interventions in real-life healthcare settings.

Objectives
- To highlight the importance of external stakeholder engagement when delivering polyvagal-informed interventions.
- To identify feasible marketing approaches for reaching target clientele for polyvagal-informed interventions.
- To explain how to present the conclusions and outcomes of polyvagal-informed interventions to different stakeholders.

> **Stakeholder Engagement in the Harmonious Body and Mind Initiative**
>
> Safe Haven Medical Clinic is a highly reputable provider of general care to patients. The healthcare leaders Dr. Reginald White (Chief Executive Officer), Dr. Stacy Jennings (Chief Clinical Officer), and Dr. Priya Cole (Chief Medical Officer) have created a three-week program called the Harmonious Body and Mind Initiative. In the program, attendees are encouraged to participate in polyvagal-informed practices. They will be provided with appropriate physical, social, and mental health resources to improve their well-being and long-term outcomes. However, despite the novelty of the healthcare intervention, there are concerns about the need to consider external stakeholder engagement.
>
> Since the program's implementation, Safe Haven has deduced that there is inadequate financial support for ensuring optimal healthcare delivery. This problem stems from the organization's failure to liaise with public and private payors, such as government health agencies and insurance companies. In addition, similar problems have emerged concerning the hospital's collaboration with other healthcare providers, learning institutions, community organizations, and advocacy groups. While these groups are crucial for the long-term implementation of the program, they have not been integrated into the service

offering. The hospital's management has also been struggling with marketing due to the difficulty of reaching the target clientele.

To resolve these challenges, Safe Haven's leaders have opted to use their clinical measures and outcomes to promote the effectiveness of the facility's polyvagal-informed interventions. Furthermore, it has become particularly crucial to create a more coherent structure for engaging with different external stakeholders involved in the program's delivery. These problems do not include the challenges faced by Safe Haven when recruiting clients from local and international areas. Even after the completion of PVT interventions, the facility's workers have been struggling to decide on appropriate measures for presenting the findings. Safe Haven's wellness initiative can be largely attributed to poor stakeholder engagement, particularly with external stakeholders.

External Stakeholder Management

The primary purpose of external stakeholder management is to allow an organization to understand how it can strategically influence its stakeholders in a manner that is positively aligned with the organization's goals. Accordingly, stakeholder management requires an organization to liaise with various types of stakeholders to ensure healthcare delivery that is in the best interests of all parties. On this note, Tampio and Ali (2022) compare stakeholder management to social inclusion, whereby an organization eliminates barriers to allow for an easy flow of information, expertise, resources, and other crucial requirements.

Understanding the relevance of a stakeholder to healthcare delivery requires healthcare leaders to follow these steps:

1. Identify the key stakeholder.
2. Understand their interests and resources.
3. Categorize them according to their characteristics.
4. Review the resulting stakeholder dynamic.
5. Develop appropriate stakeholder management strategies.

Figure 7.1 illustrates the identification and classification of healthcare stakeholders, both internal and external. The key internal stakeholders include hospital leadership and administration, medical and clinic staff, and support staff. Along with the patients, these groups have been the primary focus of the previous chapters, with the central objective of using polyvagal-informed strategies to improve employee satisfaction and patient outcomes.

However, for the implementation of polyvagal-informed mental health interventions, healthcare organizations must also consider external stakeholders: public and private payors, healthcare providers, learning and research institutions, and community organizations. Consequently, this chapter aims to reveal the best strategies for funding, collaborating with external entities, marketing, and presenting the overall findings.

Liaising with Public and Private Payors

Modern health organizations usually form agreements with different public and private payors to ensure the sustainability of their healthcare offerings. These payors have a strong influence on healthcare prices, reimbursements, and coverage policies, which highlights their dominant role over a healthcare organization's revenue streams. These payors are categorized according to their role in public and private healthcare delivery. At one end,

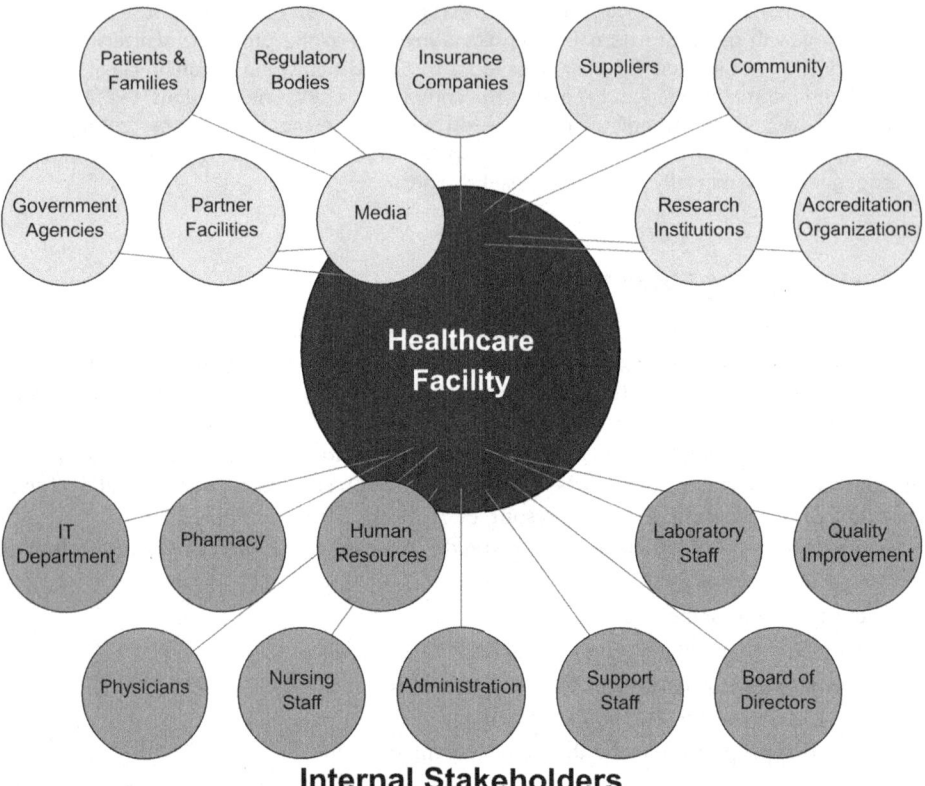

Figure 7.1 The classification of internal and external stakeholders. (Source: authors.)

public healthcare is typically funded by the government through relevant national healthcare systems (Basu et al. 2012). For that reason, public payors include government health agencies created to support the delivery of healthcare services through government-sponsored programs. These organizations include Medicaid in the United States and the National Health Service in the United Kingdom. These entities provide healthcare coverage to specific individuals, but they are subject to government regulations and oversight. Healthcare organizations that desire to implement polyvagal-informed strategies need to collaborate with the relevant agencies to leverage these interventions for the broader public. Advocacy can allow healthcare leaders to seek financial resources and support from public payors that can optimize the implementation of PVT interventions.

Conversely, private healthcare is often delivered through for-profit organizations, self-employed healthcare practitioners, and not-for-profit organizations (Basu et al. 2012). Accordingly, clients who rely on these payors often depend on private health insurance companies and self-sponsored healthcare plans. Health insurance companies are responsible for reimbursing healthcare expenses for individuals enrolled in specific insurance coverage programs. With regard to employer-sponsored health plans, most employers provide insurance coverage to their employees by deducting insurance premiums based on agreed-upon schemes.

Compared to public payors who offer services targeting low-income and disadvantaged populations, private payors usually target clients with the ability and means to enroll in customized health coverage plans. To engage with such payors, healthcare organizations need to build collaborative relationships that can encourage private payors to offer coverage beyond traditional mental health services. For instance, they can provide reimbursement that allows the facility to expand its service offerings to serve a larger client base. Overall, creating successful relationships with public and private payors can offer healthcare organizations significant rewards in supporting the implementation of polyvagal-informed interventions.

Liaising with Healthcare Providers

Another important category of external stakeholders is healthcare providers. In essence, many healthcare providers support each other in healthcare delivery to ensure comprehensive care is provided to patients. Today, collaboration between healthcare and nonhealthcare-based organizations has become a popular strategy for improving health outcomes (Alderwick et al. 2021). For instance, collaboration between general care, mental healthcare, and social services offers patients holistic care that can promote their physical, mental, emotional, and social well-being.

That said, collaboration between these groups of healthcare providers can offer an organization various opportunities for coordinating care, acquiring referrals, and sharing information. For example, primary healthcare workers tend to refer patients to mental health specialists when they feel that they do not have a complete grasp of the patient's health condition. In return, mental health workers tend to make similar referrals when they deduce that physical assessments are warranted. Through these strategies, they create interdisciplinary teams that allow them to exchange information and improve patient outcomes. Considering that the adoption of the PVT in general healthcare is still in the budding phase, healthcare providers should establish collaborations that incorporate the knowledge and expertise of multiple disciplines.

Liaising with Learning Institutions and Research Groups

As discussed earlier, the PVT is based on the contributions of several notable philosophers, such as Charles Darwin, John Hughlings Jackson, Paul MacLean, and Stephen Porges (Hays 2019). Although significant findings that support the theory have been discovered, many unresolved controversies still exist. For instance, traditional scientists and scholars categorized the ANS according to two branches, but emerging research reveals that there are three key branches that dictate autonomic responses. Therefore, continuous learning and research are crucial for understanding the strengths and flaws of different nervous system theories.

Collaborating with learning institutions can strengthen the application of PVT concepts by elucidating its limits and applications. Through educational programs, workshops, and training modules, it will be possible to disseminate fundamental knowledge concerning the

PVT. Subsequently, liaising with research groups can provide new knowledge regarding the application of the concepts in psychology, neuroscience, medicine, and biology. This interdisciplinary approach is essential for enhancing the richness of PVT concepts and ensuring the continuity of ongoing research. Therefore, collaborating with learning institutions and research groups can augment the adoption of PVT interventions by the general public.

> **Case Study 7.1: Collaborating**
>
> The situation at Safe Haven highlights the importance of collaborating with public and private payors to improve the sustainability of the Harmonious Body and Mind Initiative. Public payors can be used to support clients from low-income and disadvantaged backgrounds, while private payors can offer resources and funding for employed clients with special mental health needs.
>
> With regard to collaborations with healthcare providers, the facility needs to establish mechanisms for delivering holistic care that focuses on physical, mental, and emotional well-being. In addition, Safe Haven should also establish solid relationships with learning institutions and research organizations. These parties can strengthen the depth of PVT knowledge, thereby increasing their applications in diverse clinical settings. Collaboration with these stakeholders can allow Safe Haven to expand its coverage beyond traditional mental health services and increase the reach of PVT interventions.

Marketing Polyvagal-Informed Interventions

The implementation of polyvagal-informed strategies requires an organization to have a laser focus on the target clientele. In this case, the interventions are designed for individuals struggling with mild, moderate, or severe distress due to a specific cause. The root cause may be work stressors, anxiety, depression, or trauma. Thus, healthcare providers need to use appropriate strategies to identify these individuals and recruit them to the program.

When the target is local clients, the most effective strategy is to leverage community-specific channels, including local media, community-based organizations, and community events. The organization can use traditional marketing strategies, such as the distribution of posters, broadcasting on radio and television stations, and seeking word-of-mouth referrals. These channels can allow a healthcare provider to recruit clients who are eligible for the program and are within the facility's vicinity.

However, when targeting clients in the international landscape, organizations are recommended to use online channels, including social media, websites, and online ads. Digital marketing can allow the facility to reach a greater number of patients, who will then be directed to enroll in the mental health program. These channels offer a tailored strategy for reaching clients with imbalances in their mind–body connection.

> **Case Study 7.2: Reaching the Market**
>
> The leaders at Safe Haven are facing a dilemma regarding the best strategy for recruiting clients. Although the PVT interventions can be adopted by a wide variety of patients, it is particularly effective for patients with abnormal shifts in their ANS.
>
> Identifying these individuals can be exceedingly challenging in real-life scenarios. Therefore, the clinic's leaders are encouraged to employ multiple marketing strategies.

Posters, TV ads, and radio ads can be used to reach eligible clients in the facility's vicinity. Afterward, social media and websites can be used to display relevant content concerning the requirements, procedures, and outcomes of PVT interventions. These two approaches can cause a surge in the number of patients enrolling in the Harmonious Body and Mind Initiative.

Incorporating Data from Clinical Measures

Healthcare providers and scholars who take part in research also need to present their findings in research studies or conferences to demonstrate their validity. For that reason, the quality measures for assessing the outcomes of polyvagal-informed interventions need to be comprehensive to promote the adoption of PVT concepts in diverse healthcare settings. For instance, Chapter 5 offers a list of clinical measures that can be utilized to acquire comprehensive results regarding the outcomes of polyvagal-informed strategies.

Among the clinical measures, subjective measures and behavioral observation are inherently suitable for explaining the qualitative findings because the results are based on the participants' or observers' opinions. Alternatively, objective measures and standardized psychological tests can be utilized to provide quantitative metrics regarding the outcomes of PVT interventions. These instruments are designed to benchmark specific states and characteristics (stress, trauma, depression, anxiety, wellness, perceived safety, body awareness, and social engagement) that are commonly associated with the PVT. The presentation of these clinical findings in studies and conferences can emphasize the effectiveness of polyvagal-informed interventions in real-life clinical settings.

> **Case Study 7.3: Collecting the Data**
>
> The Harmonious Body and Mind Initiative is an innovative PVT therapy, but its efficacy will remain uncertain until the healthcare providers at Safe Haven report the intervention's findings. That said, the leaders can utilize a mix of qualitative and quantitative measures to describe the outcomes of the therapy.
>
> The subjective scales and behavioral observations can offer essential insights into the perceptions and opinions of the participants, while the objective measures and standardized psychological measures offer a more calculatable understanding of a patient's health outcomes. By presenting these findings, the leaders at Safe Haven can create awareness regarding the potential applications of PVT interventions in the healthcare industry and other professional sectors.

Key Takeaways

- The success of PVT interventions depends on the input of not only internal stakeholders but also external stakeholders because they tend to have significant investment in healthcare ventures. That said, stakeholder engagement is a social inclusion process that allows healthcare organizations to interact with different stakeholders and create solid relationships to support the flow of information, expertise, and resources. The process begins with identifying the stakeholders and understanding their interests. With a firm understanding of their characteristics and dynamics, it will be possible to implement suitable management strategies for interacting with stakeholders. For instance, public and private payors play a vital role in ensuring the financial stability of healthcare undertakings, while support from other healthcare providers provides an interdisciplinary approach to delivering holistic care to patients. In comparison, liaising with learning institutions and research groups can create opportunities for expanding the scope of knowledge regarding PVT interventions.

- Identifying suitable clients who are eligible for PVT interventions can be a significant obstacle. Accordingly, the most effective recommendation is to employ marketing tactics that cover local communities as well as the international market. For local clientele, healthcare providers can leverage community-specific channels that will allow them to reach target clients in close proximity. Consequently, the introduction of online marketing channels can complement these measures by increasing the geographic reach of marketing efforts.
- Another approach that can strengthen the adoption of PVT interventions is the presentation of its findings in research studies and relevant conferences. These studies and conferences are often used to disseminate essential healthcare knowledge to different groups. Nonetheless, without valid and reliable findings, some groups may struggle to understand the practicality of the PVT interventions. To address this problem, healthcare leaders are encouraged to rely on a combination of qualitative and quantitative measures (see Chapter 5). With this knowledge, healthcare organizations that utilize PVT concepts can demonstrate their effectiveness and enhance their integration into diverse healthcare practices.

Conclusion

The PVT, as developed by Stephen Porges, has a profound impact on how we understand the human ANS and our emphasis on staying safe and connected with others. Although having been adopted in behavioral health circles, the theory is just beginning to break ground in terms of how we view other clinical specialties (such as primary care), as well as nonclinical aspects of healthcare.

As we have reviewed in this book, PVT concepts can be applied to help us become better leaders, managers, and healthcare team members. By introducing the core concepts of this theory and exploring how they might be helpful in these various aspects of running a healthcare organization, we hope you will have gained some new ideas and tools. Ultimately, the goal is to help reduce stress and burnout in staff, improve clinical outcomes in patients, and reduce overall costs by reducing staff turnover and lengths of stay for patients (in hospital services).

We hope you found this book both interesting and stimulating and that it helps you to innovate ways to improve lives. If you are interested in more detailed, experiential training, and support, NeuroConsulting Group offers online (on demand and live) and in-person consulting and training. Whether you want to build skills or assist in implementing the PVT into your healthcare organization, visit https://neuroconsultinggroup.com for more information.

References

Abi-Esber, N., Brooks, A. W., & Burris, E. (2022). Feeling seen: Leader eye gaze promotes psychological safety, participation, and voice. Harvard Business School Working Paper.

Aga, D. A. (2016). Transactional leadership and project success: The moderating role of goal clarity. *Procedia Computer Science, 100,* 517–525.

Ahmed, R., Ucci, M., Mumovic, D., & Bagkeris, E. (2022). Effects of thermal sensation and acclimatization on cognitive performance of adult female students in Saudi Arabia using multivariable-multilevel statistical modeling. *Indoor Air, 32*(2), e13005.

Alarcón-Espinoza, M., Sanduvete-Chaves, S., Anguera, M. T., Samper García, P., & Chacón-Moscoso, S. (2022). Emotional self-regulation in everyday life: A systematic review. *Frontiers in Psychology, 13,* 884756.

Alderwick, H., Hutchings, A., Briggs, A., & Mays, N. (2021). The impacts of collaboration between local health care and non-health care organizations and factors shaping how they work: A systematic review of reviews. *BMC Public Health, 21,* 1–16.

American Psychological Association. (2017). PTSD assessment instruments. American Psychological Association. www.apa.org/ptsd-guideline/assessment.

Arany, L., & Popovics, P. (2022). The modern leader: The history of leadership styles and the most important qualities of a modern leader. *Cross-Cultural Management Journal, 24*(2), 91.

Awada, M., Becerik-Gerber, B., Liu, R., et al. (2023). Ten questions concerning the impact of environmental stress on office workers, *Building and Environment, 229,* 109964. https://doi.org/10.1016/j.buildenv.2022.109964.

Bacon, B. (2013). Intuitive intelligence in leadership. *Management Services, 57*(3), 26–29.

Bae, S., & Choi, M. (2023). Age and workplace ageism: A systematic review and meta-analysis. *Journal of Gerontological Social Work, 66*(6), 724–738.

Banks, G. C., McCauley, K. D., Gardner, W. L., & Guler, C. E. (2016). A meta-analytic review of authentic and transformational leadership: A test for redundancy. *The Leadership Quarterly, 27*(4), 634–652.

Barratt, B. B. (2010). Psychology at the crossroads. In B. B. Barratt (Ed.), *The emergence of somatic psychology and bodymind therapy* (pp. 7–21). Palgrave Macmillan UK.

Basu, S., Andrews, J., Kishore, S., Panjabi, R., & Stuckler, D. (2012). Comparative performance of private and public healthcare systems in low-and middle-income countries: A systematic review. *PLoS Medicine, 9*(6), e1001244.

Berry, D., & Bell, M. P. (2012). Inequality in organizations: Stereotyping, discrimination, and labor law exclusions. *Equality, Diversity and Inclusion: An International Journal, 31*(3), 236–248.

Bhui, K., Dinos, S., Galant-Miecznikowska, M., de Jongh, B., & Stansfeld, S. (2016). Perceptions of work stress causes and effective interventions in employees working in public, private and non-governmental organisations: A qualitative study. *BJPsych Bulletin, 40*(6), 318–325.

Blume, C., Garbazza, C., & Spitschan, M. (2019). Effects of light on human circadian rhythms, sleep and mood. *Somnologie, 23*(3), 147.

Brazie, R., & Vanderpal, G. (2023). *The steadfast leader.* McGraw Hill.

Brown, R., & Gerbarg, P. L. (2012). *The healing power of the breath: Simple techniques to reduce stress and anxiety, enhance concentration, and balance your emotions.* Shambhala Publications.

Campbell, P. D., Miller, A. M., & Woesner, M. E. (2017). Bright light therapy: Seasonal affective disorder and beyond. *The Einstein Journal of Biology and Medicine, 32*, E13.

Chappuis, C., & Grandjean, D. (2022). Set the tone: Trustworthy and dominant novel voices classification using explicit judgement and machine learning techniques. *PLoS ONE, 17*(6), e0267432.

Choi, S. L., Goh, C. F., Adam, M. B. H., & Tan, O. K. (2016). Transformational leadership, empowerment, and job satisfaction: The mediating role of employee empowerment. *Human Resources for Health, 14*(1), 1–14.

Cooper, L. (2020, July 30). Your healing voice: The benefits of singing for health and well-being. The British Academy of Sound Therapy. https://britishacademyofsoundtherapy.com/research/singing-for-health/.

Couvy-Duchesne, B., Davenport, T. A., Martin, N. G., Wright, M. J., & Hickie, I. B. (2017). Validation and psychometric properties of the Somatic and Psychological HEalth REport (SPHERE) in a young Australian-based population sample using non-parametric item response theory. *BMC Psychiatry, 17*(1), 1–24.

Crandall, R. E., & Crandall, W. R. (2008). *New methods of competing in the global marketplace: Critical success factors from service and manufacturing.* CRC Press.

Cui, J., Li, M., Wei, Y., et al. (2022). Inhalation aromatherapy via brain-targeted nasal delivery: Natural volatiles or essential oils on mood disorders. *Frontiers in Pharmacology, 13*, 860043.

Dana, D. (2018). *The polyvagal theory in therapy: Engaging the rhythm of regulation* (Norton Series on Interpersonal Neurobiology). W. W. Norton & Company.

Dana, D. (2020). *Polyvagal exercises for safety and connection: 50 client-centered practices* (Norton Series on Interpersonal Neurobiology). W. W. Norton & Company.

Dana, D. (2023). *Polyvagal practices: Anchoring the self in safety.* W. W. Norton & Company.

Daumeyer, N. M., Onyeador, I. N., Brown, X., & Richeson, J. A. (2019). Consequences of attributing discrimination to implicit vs. explicit bias. *Journal of Experimental Social Psychology, 84*, 103812.

Deal, J. (2019, July 31). A hierarchy model for leadership development. *Medium.* https://medium.com/swlh/a-hierarchy-model-for-leadership-development-cee911071e4a.

Eswaran, V. (2021, July 22). Don't underestimate the power of silence. *Harvard Business Review.* https://hbr.org/2021/07/dont-underestimate-the-power-of-silence.

Ezhumalai, S., Muralidhar, D., Dhanasekarapandian, R., & Nikketha, B. S. (2018). Group interventions. *Indian Journal of Psychiatry, 60*(Suppl 4), S514.

Flarity, K., Gentry, J. E., & Mesnikoft, N. (2013). The effectiveness of an educational program on preventing and treating compassion fatigue in emergency nurses. *Advanced Emergency Nursing Journal. 35*(3), 247–258.

Gardner, R. (2023, September 8). 12 types of organizational culture you should know. AIHR. www.aihr.com/blog/types-of-organizational-culture/.

Ghazzawi, K., Shoughari, R. E., & Osta, B. E. (2017). Situational leadership and its effectiveness in rising employee productivity: A study on North Lebanon organization. *Human Resource Management Research, 7*(3), 102–110.

Goldsby, T. L., Goldsby, M. E., McWalters, M., & Mills, P. J. (2022). Sound healing: Mood, emotional, and spiritual well-being interrelationships. *Religions, 13*(2), 123.

Guarnera, M., Hichy, Z., Cascio, M. I., & Carrubba, S. (2015). Facial expressions and ability to recognize emotions from eyes or mouth in children. *Europe's Journal of Psychology, 11*(2), 183.

Hamill, R. W., Shapiro, R. E., & Vizzard, M. A. (2012). Peripheral autonomic nervous system. In D. Robertson, I. Biaggioni, P. A. Low, G. Burnstock, & J. F. R. Paton (Eds.), *Primer on the autonomic nervous system* (3rd ed.) (pp. 17–26). Academic Press.

Hays, S. (2019). Nature as discourse: Transdisciplinarity and vagus nerve function. *Transdisciplinary Journal of Engineering & Science, 10*, 18–27.

Hunt, T., & Fedynich, L. (2019). Leadership: Past, present, and future – An evolution of an idea. *Journal of Arts and Humanities, 8*(2), 22–26.

Jensen, U. T., Andersen, L. B., Bro, L. L., et al. (2016). Conceptualizing and measuring transformational and transactional leadership. *Administration and Society, 51*(1), 3–33.

Jogdand, A. M. (2022). Color therapy in mental health and well-being. *International Journal of Creative Research Thoughts (IJCRT), 10*(1), a124–a130.

Kamphaus, R. W., & Tsushima, W. T. (2016). Behavioral observations and assessment. In J. C. Norcross, G. R. VandenBos, D. K. Freedheim, B. O. Olatunji, & R. Krishnamurthy (Eds.), *APA Handbook of Clinical Psychology: Vol. 2* (pp. 17–29). American Psychological Association.

Kaplan, R., Kaplan, S., & Ryan, R. L. (1998). *With people in mind: Design and management of everyday nature.* Washington, DC: Island Press

Kawai, H., Kishimoto, M., Okahisa, Y., Sakamoto, S., Terada, S., & Takaki, M. (2023). Initial outcomes of the safe and sound protocol on patients with adult autism spectrum disorder: Exploratory pilot study. *International Journal of Environmental Research and Public Health, 20*(6), 4862.

Ke, M. H., Hsieh, K. T., & Hsieh, W. Y. (2022). Effects of aromatherapy on the physical and mental health and pressure of the middle-aged and elderly in the community. *Applied Sciences, 12*(10), 4823.

Khalsa, S. S., Adolphs, R., Cameron, O. G., et al. (2018). Interoception and mental health: A roadmap. *Biological Psychiatry: Cognitive Neuroscience and Neuroimaging, 3*(6), 501–513.

Khan, H., Rehmat, M., Butt, T. H., Farooqi, S., & Asim, J. (2020). Impact of transformational leadership on work performance, burnout and social loafing: A mediation model. *Future Business Journal, 6*(1), 1–13.

Khosravi, M., Haqbin, A., Zare, Z., et al. (2012). Selecting the most suitable organizational structure for hospitals: An integrated fuzzy FUCOM-MARCOS method. *Cost Effectiveness and Resource Allocation, 20*, 29. https://doi.org/10.1186/s12962-022-00362-3.

Kim, D. H. (2016). Emergency preparedness and the development of health care coalitions: A dynamic process. *Nursing Clinics, 51*(4), 545–554.

Kim, E. S., Chen, Y., Nakamura, J. S., Ryff, C. D., & VanderWeele, T. J. (2022). Sense of purpose in life and subsequent physical, behavioral, and psychosocial health: An outcome-wide approach. *American Journal of Health Promotion, 36*(1), 137–147.

Kim, J., & Jung, H. S. (2022). The effect of employee competency and organizational culture on employees' perceived stress for better workplace. *International Journal of Environmental Research and Public Health, 19*(8), 4428.

Knowles, R. (2023, December 12). Dr. Stephen Porges' latest publication on the Polyvagal theory. Unyte Integrated Listening. http://bit.ly/4mustvm.

Koslouski, J. B., Wilson-Mendenhall, C. D., Parsafar, P., Goldberg, S., Martin, M. Y., & Chafouleas, S. M. (2022). Measuring emotional well-being through subjective report: A scoping review of reviews. *BMJ Open, 12*(12), 1–9.

Kroll, E., Veit, S., & Ziegler, M. (2021). The discriminatory potential of modern recruitment trends – A mixed-method study from Germany. *Frontiers in Psychology, 12*, 634376.

Kuhfuß, M., Maldei, T., Hetmanek, A., & Baumann, N. (2021). Somatic experiencing – effectiveness and key factors of a body-oriented trauma therapy: A scoping literature review. *European Journal of Psychotraumatology, 12*(1), 1929023.

Kwon, M., & Remøy, H. (2020). Office employee satisfaction: The influence of design factors on psychological user satisfaction. *Facilities, 38*(1/2), 1–19.

Lancee, B. (2021). Ethnic discrimination in hiring: Comparing groups across contexts. Results from a cross-national field experiment. *Journal of Ethnic and Migration Studies, 47*(6), 1181–1200.

Langley-Brady, D. L., Shutes, J., Vinson, J. J., & Zadinsky, J. K. (2023). Aromatherapy through the lens of trauma-informed care: Stress-reduction practices for healthcare professionals. *Journal of Interprofessional Education & Practice*, *30*, 100602.

Lobel, T. (2016). *Sensation: The new science of physical intelligence*. Atria Books.

LoBue, V., Baker, L., & Thrasher, C. (2017). Through the eyes of a child: Preschoolers' identification of emotional expressions from the child affective facial expression (CAFE) set. *Cognition and Emotion*, *32*(5), 1122–1130.

Lucas, A. R., Klepin, H. D., Porges, S. W., & Rejeski, W. J. (2021). Mindfulness-based movement: A polyvagal perspective. In S. W. Porges (Ed.), *Polyvagal safety: Attachment, communication, self-regulation* (pp. 77–87). W. W. Norton & Company.

Lukan, J., Bolliger, L., Pauwels, N. S., Luštrek, M., Bacquer, D. D., & Clays, E. (2022). Work environment risk factors causing day-to-day stress in occupational settings: A systematic review. *BMC Public Health*, *22*(1), 240.

Lyons, J. B., & Schneider, T. R. (2009). The effects of leadership style on stress outcomes. *The Leadership Quarterly*, *20*(5), 737–748.

Marmarosh, C. L., Sandage, S., Wade, N., Captari, L. E., & Crabtree, S. (2022). New horizons in group psychotherapy research and practice from third wave positive psychology: A practice-friendly review. *Research in Psychotherapy: Psychopathology, Process, and Outcome*, *25*(3), 643.

McFarlane, A. C., McKenzie, D. P., Van Hooff, M., & Browne, D. (2008). Somatic and psychological dimensions of screening for psychiatric morbidity: A community validation of the SPHERE Questionnaire. *Journal of Psychosomatic Research*, *65*(4), 337–345.

Menefee, D. S., Ledoux, T., & Johnston, C. A. (2022). The importance of emotional regulation in mental health. *American Journal of Lifestyle Medicine*, *16*(1), 28–31.

Michailidou, F., Bearth, A., Deilmann, C., & Siegrist, M. (2023). Scent and sustainability: Investigating consumer evaluations of biocatalysis and naturalness in fragrances. *Food Quality and Preference*, *111*, 104994.

Miles, A., & Sadler-Smith, E. (2014). "With recruitment I always feel I need to listen to my gut": The role of intuition in employee selection. *Personnel Review*, *43*(4), 606–627.

Miller, L. A., & Lovler, R. L. (2018). *Foundations of psychological testing: A practical approach*. Sage Publications.

Moon, E., Yang, M., Seon, Q., & Linnaranta, O. (2021). Relevance of objective measures in psychiatric disorders: Rest-activity rhythm and psychophysiological measures. *Current Psychiatry Reports*, *23*(12), 85.

Morganstein, J. C., West, J. C., & Ursano, R. J. (2017). Work-associated trauma. In K. J. Brower & M. B. Riba (Eds.), *Physician mental health and well-being: Research and practice* (pp. 33–60). Springer.

Nieto-Rodriguez, A. (2023). A new approach to writing job descriptions. *Harvard Business Review*. https://hbr.org/2023/10/a-new-approach-to-writing-job-descriptions.

Odumeru, J. A., & Ogbonna, I. G. (2013). Transformational vs. transactional leadership theories: Evidence in literature. *International Review of Management and Business Research*, *2*(2), 355.

Okechukwu, C. A., Souza, K., Davis, K. D., & De Castro, A. B. (2014). Discrimination, harassment, abuse, and bullying in the workplace: Contribution of workplace injustice to occupational health disparities. *American Journal of Industrial Medicine*, *57*(5), 573–586.

Parent, J. D., & Lovelace, K. J. (2018). Employee engagement, positive organizational culture and individual adaptability. *On the Horizon*, *26*(3), 206–214.

Plant Therapy. (2019, February 1). Fragrance wheel. www.planttherapy.com/blogs/blog/shop-by-scent-the-fragrance-wheel.

Platt, M. (2020). *The leader's brain: Enhance your leadership, build stronger teams, make better decisions, and inspire greater innovation with neuroscience*. University of Pennsylvania Press.

Poli, A., Gemignani, A., Soldani, F., & Miccoli, M. (2021). A systematic review of a polyvagal perspective on embodied contemplative practices as promoters of cardiorespiratory coupling and traumatic stress recovery for PTSD and OCD: Research methodologies and state of the art. *International Journal of Environmental Research and Public Health, 18*(22), 11778.

Polyvagal Institute. (n.d.). Assessments. www.polyvagalinstitute.org/assessments.

Porges, S. W. (2003). The polyvagal theory: Phylogenetic contributions to social behavior. *Physiology & Behavior, 79*(3), 503–513.

Porges, S. W. (2007). The polyvagal perspective. *Biological Psychology, 74*(2), 116–143.

Porges, S. W. (2011). *The polyvagal theory: Neurophysiological foundations of emotions, attachment, communication, and self-regulation* (Norton Series on Interpersonal Neurobiology). W. W. Norton & Company.

Porges, S. W. (2015). Making the world safe for our children: Down-regulating defence and up-regulating social engagement to "optimise" the human experience. *Children Australia, 40*(2), 114–123.

Porges, S. W. (2021a). *Polyvagal safety: Attachment, communication, self-regulation (IPNB)*. W. W. Norton & Company.

Porges, S. W. (2021b). Polyvagal theory: A biobehavioral journey to sociality. *Comprehensive Psychoneuroendocrinology, 7*, 100069.

Porges, S. W. (2022). Polyvagal theory: A science of safety. *Frontiers in Integrative Neuroscience, 16*, 871227.

Porges, S. W., & Kolacz, J. (2021). Neurocardiology through the lens of the polyvagal theory: Mindfulness-based movement – A polyvagal perspective. In S. W. Porges (Ed.), *Polyvagal safety: Attachment, communication, self-regulation* (pp. 77–87). W. W. Norton & Company.

Potter, D., & Starke, J. (2022). *Building a culture of conscious leadership*. Taylor & Francis.

Price, C. J., & Hooven, C. (2018). Interoceptive awareness skills for emotion regulation: Theory and approach of mindful awareness in body-oriented therapy (MABT). *Frontiers in Psychology, 9*, 798.

Reihl, K. M., Hurley, R. A., & Taber, K. H. (2015). Neurobiology of implicit and explicit bias: Implications for clinicians. *The Journal of Neuropsychiatry and Clinical Neurosciences, 27*(4), A6-253.

Reuille-Dupont, S. (2020). Applications of somatic psychology: Movement and body experience in the treatment of dissociative disorders. *Body, Movement and Dance in Psychotherapy, 16*(2), 105–119.

Rink, L. C., Oyesanya, T. O., Adair, K. C., Humphreys, J. C., Silva, S. G., & Sexton, J. B. (2023). Stressors among healthcare workers: A summative content analysis. *Global Qualitative Nursing Research, 10*, 23333936231161127.

Roscigno, V. J. (2019). Discrimination, sexual harassment, and the impact of workplace power. *Socius, 5*, 2378023119853894.

Roxberg, Å., Tryselius, K., Gren, M., et al. (2020). Space and place for health and care. *International Journal of Qualitative Studies on Health and Well-being, 15*(sup1), 1750263.

Rozario, S. D., Venkatraman, S., & Abbas, A. (2019). Challenges in recruitment and selection process: An empirical study. *Challenges, 10*(2), 35.

Sánchez-López, M. T., Fernández-Berrocal, P., Gómez-Leal, R., & Megías-Robles, A. (2022). Evidence on the relationship between emotional intelligence and risk behavior: A systematic and meta-analytic review. *Frontiers in Psychology, 13*, 810012.

Schoen, S. A., Miller, L. J., & Sullivan, J. C. (2014). Measurement in sensory modulation: The sensory processing scale assessment. *The American Journal of Occupational Therapy, 68*(5), 522–530.

Seijts, G. H., & Gandz, J. (2018). Transformational change and leader character. *Business Horizons, 61*(2), 239–249.

Shapiro, F. (2014). The role of eye movement desensitization and reprocessing (EMDR) therapy in medicine: Addressing the psychological and physical symptoms stemming from adverse life experiences. *The Permanente Journal, 18*(1), 71–77.

Sherrington, C. S. (1906). *The integrative action of the nervous system*. Yale University Press.

Specchia, M. L., Cozzolino, M. R., Carini, E., Di Pilla, A., Galletti, C., Ricciardi, W., & Damiani, G. (2021). Leadership styles and nurses' job satisfaction: Results of a systematic review. *International Journal of Environmental Research and Public Health, 18*(4), 1552.

Stamarski, C. S., & Son Hing, L. S. (2015). Gender inequalities in the workplace: The effects of organizational structures, processes, practices, and decision makers' sexism. *Frontiers in Psychology, 6*, 1400.

Starcke, K., & Brand, M. (2012). Decision making under stress: A selective review. *Neuroscience & Biobehavioral Reviews, 36*(4), 1228–1248.

Sun, Y., Fu, Z., Bo, Q., Mao, Z., Ma, X., & Wang, C. (2020). The reliability and validity of PHQ-9 in patients with major depressive disorder in psychiatric hospital. *BMC Psychiatry, 20*, 1–7.

Tampio, K., Haapasalo, H., & Ali, F. (2022). Stakeholder analysis and landscape in a hospital project: Elements and implications for value creation. *International Journal of Managing Projects in Business, 15*(8), 48–76.

TCP Lighting. (2017, Dec 12). The psychological impact of light & color. www.tcpi.com/psychological-impact-light-color/.

Thomas, O., & Reimann, O. (2023). The bias blind spot among HR employees in hiring decisions. *German Journal of Human Resource Management, 37*(1), 5–22.

Thompson, G., & Glasø, L. (2018). Situational leadership theory: A test from a leader-follower congruence approach. *Leadership & Organization Development Journal, 39*(5), 574–591.

Thornicroft, G., & Slade, M. (2014). New trends in assessing the outcomes of mental health interventions. *World Psychiatry, 13*(2), 118–124.

VandenBussche, S., & Hokkanen, A. (2021, February 8). Culturally reflective health care buildings. *Health Facilities Management Magazine.* www.hfmmagazine.com/articles/4098-culturally-reflective-health-care-buildings.

Vanderpal, G., & Brazie, R. (2022). Exploratory study of polyvagal theory and underlying stress and trauma that influence major leadership approaches. *Journal of Applied Business and Economics, 24*(1), 205–230.

Vanderpal, G., & Brazie, R. (2022). Influence of basic human behaviors (influenced by brain architecture and function), and past traumatic events on investor behavior and financial bias. *Journal of Accounting and Finance, 22*(3), 33–53.

Watt, G. V. D., & Janca, A. (2008). Aromatherapy in nursing and mental health care. *Contemporary Nurse, 30*(1), 69–75.

West, J., Liang, B., & Spinazzola, J. (2017). Trauma sensitive yoga as a complementary treatment for posttraumatic stress disorder: A qualitative descriptive analysis. *International Journal of Stress Management, 24*(2), 173.

Whatling, E. (2020). Stress and management. *Crisis Response Journal.* www.crisis-response.com/Articles/593147/Stress_and_crisis.aspx.

Whittington, J. L. (2017). Creating a positive organization through servant leadership. In C. J. Davis (Ed.), *Servant leadership and followership: Examining the impact on workplace behavior* (pp. 51–80). Springer.

Winston, B., & Fields, D. (2015). Seeking and measuring the essential behaviors of servant leadership. *Leadership & Organization Development Journal, 36*(4), 413–434.

Winter, M., & Tyree, K. (2021). Polyvagal theory. In T. K. Shackelford & V. A. Weekes-Shackelford (Eds.), *Encyclopedia of evolutionary psychological science* (pp. 6062–6066). Springer.

Wolgast, S., Bäckström, M., & Björklund, F. (2017). Tools for fairness: Increased structure in the selection process reduces discrimination. *PLoS One, 12*(12), e0189512

Yang, X. Y., Yang, N. B., Huang, F. F., Ren, S., & Li, Z. J. (2021). Effectiveness of acupuncture on anxiety disorder: A systematic review and meta-analysis of randomised controlled trials. *Annals of General Psychiatry, 20*(1), 1–14.

Zeng, E., Dong, Y., Yan, L., & Lin, A. (2022). Perceived safety in the neighborhood: Exploring the role of built environment, social factors, physical activity and multiple pathways of influence. *Buildings, 13*(1), 2.

Index

acoustic comfort, 47
acupuncture, 43
acute risk and crisis (PVT)
   body position, 59
   eye contact, 59
   overview, 58–59
   tone of voice, 59
affinity bias, 63
ageism, discrimination, 68
amygdala, 18
appraisal bias, 63
aromatherapy
   case study, 45–46
   fragrance wheel, 44
   inhalation mechanisms, 44–45
   mood regulation, 44
   triggering autonomic responses, 43–44
attributional bias, 63
autonomic nervous system (ANS)
   divisions, 8, 10
   mapping, 33–37
   physiological and behavioral states, 4–5
   protection and connection baseline, 66
   regulation strategies exercises, 26–28
   safety and, 5
   social engagement system, 9, 11
   unconscious automated processes, 9
autonomic nervous system (ANS), functional states
   dorsal vagal state, 13
   sympathetic state, 13
   ventral vagal state, 13

behavioral observation
   case study, 104
   overview, 103–104
   pros and cons, 104
bias and discrimination, HRM talent management
   forms of, 62
   impact of, 61–62
   pressures and stresses, 60

bias mitigation steps, polyvagal-informed
   candidate baseline matching, 66–68
   case study, 67–68, 69
   challenges of, 65–66
   potential inequalities matching, 68–69
body language (PVT), 51
Brain-Body Center Sensory Scale, 106
bright light therapy, 46

central nervous system (CNS) and neuroception, 100
cognitive bias, 65–66
complementary and alternative medicines (CAM), 44
confirmation bias, 63
conformity bias, 63
connection state (ANS), 66
contrast effect, 63

Darwin, Charles, 6–7
demeanor (PVT), 52
dorsal vagal complex (DVC)
   location and function, 8
   overview, 28
dorsal vagal state
   challenge activities, 57–58
   challenge comments, 56
   change activities, 57
   change comments, 55
   definition, 13
   employment candidates, 67
   exercises, 25–26
   polyvagal ladder, 14
   stay activities, 56–57
   stay comments, 55

education (PVT), 32–33
embodied cognition, 12
emotional well-being metric, 102–103
environmental psychology, 113
expectation anchor, 63
explicit bias, 62
eye contact (PVT), 50

eye movement desensitization and reprocessing (EMDR), 42–43

facial expressions (PVT), 50–51
fight-or-flight response, 8
first-impression bias, 63

gender-based discrimination, 69
Generalized Anxiety Disorder-7 (GAD-7), 106
Glimmers and Triggers Map, 34–35
group interventions (PVT), 48–49

halo effect, 63
health, definition, 99
health scales and measures
   anxiety scales, 106
   body awareness and perception measures, 106
   case study, 107
   depression scales, 105–106
   overview, 107–108
   safety and social engagement measures, 106
   sensory processing measures, 106
   Somatic and Psychological Health Report (SPHERE), 105
   stress scales, 105
   well-being and life satisfaction measures, 106
healthcare environment design
   example, 109–110
   safety and, 110
healthcare environment design, important considerations
   emergency preparedness, 112
   enhancing surroundings, 111
   nature, 112
   private spaces, 112
   safety, 111–113

Index 133

social and cultural
  diversity, 112
welcoming
  environment, 111
healthcare environment
  design, workplace layouts
environmental
  psychology, 113
  visual appeal, 113–116
horn effect, 63
human resources management
  (HRM), talent recruitment
  bias mitigation steps, 65–71
  common biases, 62–63
  job description accuracy,
    71–72
  recruitment bias and
    discrimination, 60–62
  supportive organizational
    culture creation, 72–74
hypothalamic-pituitary-
  adrenal (HPA) axis, 18

immobilization state. *see* dorsal
  vagal state
implicit bias, 62
in-group bias, 63
interoception
  body awareness and
    perception measures, 106
  conscious awareness of
    physiological reactions, 12
  definition, 11
  development importance, 29
  embodied cognition, 12
  history, 11
intuitive decision-making
  definition, 89
  steadfast leadership and,
    89

Jackson, John Hughlings, 7

language of design (PVT), 52
leadership, characteristics for
  effective
  ANS attunement, 90–91
  eight behaviors of, 90
  example, 75
  social brain network
    and, 90
  team chemistry, 91
leadership styles, healthcare
  background, 78
  definition, 78

healthcare organization type
  and, 80
hierarchy model of
  development, 78–79
importance of, 78
servant leadership, 86–88
situational leadership,
  84–86
steadfast leadership, 88–90
summary, 96
transactional leadership,
  80–82
transformational leadership,
  83–84
light therapy, 46
lighting, environmental
  safety and, 111–112
  visual appeal, 113–114

Maclean, Paul, 7
mapping (ANS)
  case study, 37
  Glimmers and Triggers Map,
    34–35
  group, 33
  Personal Profile Map,
    33–34
  reasons for, 33
  Regulating Resources Map,
    36–37
mobilization state. *see*
  sympathetic state
"moments between" awareness
  skill, 92
music of the voice, 47

nervous system
  Darwin on, 6–7
  Jackson on, 7
  Maclean on, 7
neuroception
  defensive strategy
    downregulation, 11
  definition, 9
  emotional regulation
    and, 100
  exercises, 18–21
  Porges on, 9
Neuroception of Psychological
  Safety Scale, 106
nociception, 9

objective measures, healthcare
  outcomes
  background, 101

case study, 102
pros and cons, 101
summary, 101
organizational culture
  development
  case study, 74
  challenges of, 73
  definition, 72
  polyvagal-informed steps, 73
  types of, 72–73
ostrich effect, 65
overconfidence bias, 63

parasympathetic nervous
  system (PNS),
  components
  dorsal vagal complex
    (DVC), 8
  ventral vagal complex
    (VVC), 8
parasympathetic nervous
  system (PNS),
  schematic, 10
Patient Health Questionnaire-9
  (PHQ-9), 105
personal containment skill, 92
Personal Profile Map, 33–34
physical proximity (PVT),
  51–52
polyvagal ladder
  example, 15–16
  overview, 13–15, 29
  Personal Profile Map, 33–34
Polyvagal Promotions
  Protocol, approaches
  activities, 56–58
  comments, 54, 55
  patient family members, 58
Polyvagal Promotions
  Protocol, stages
  challenge, 55–56
  change, 55
  stay, 54–55
polyvagal theory
  ANS shifts, 4–5
  ANS states, 5
  definition, 4
  healthcare leadership, 75
  healthcare relevance, 6
  human resource
    management (HRM),
    60–74
  mammalian evolutionary
    transition, 5
  safety science and, 5

Index

polyvagal theory, core concepts
  ANS functional states, 12–13
  importance of, 28–29
  major divisions of ANS, 8–9
  neuroception and interoception, 9–12
  polyvagal ladder, 13–15
polyvagal theory, healthcare contributions
  ANS practical techniques, 17
  example, 17
  overview, 29
  stress and trauma, 16–17
polyvagal theory, healthcare contributions to
  history, 16
  medical advances, 16
  skills for high-stress environment, 91–93
  somatic psychology, 16
polyvagal theory, healthcare integration
  body–mind connection, 31
  bridge between cognitive and somatic perspectives, 31, 59
  challenge of, 31–32
  reasons for, 31
polyvagal theory, healthcare integration steps
  ANS mapping, 33–37
  education, 32–33
  interoception strengthening, 39–42
  polyvagal-informed interventions, 42–48
  self-regulation skills, 37–39
polyvagal theory, history
  early 1900s, 7
  founding fathers, 6–7
  Porges's theory, 7–8
polyvagal theory (PVT), healthcare outcomes measurement
  background, 100
  behavioral observation, 103–104
  case study, 98–99
  challenges of, 99–100
  objective measures, 101–102
  standardized psychological assessments, 104–107
  subjective measures, 102–103
  summary, 107–108
polyvagal-informed interventions
  acupuncture, 43
  aromatherapy, 43–46
  case study, 47–48
  definition, 5
  eye movement desensitization and reprocessing (EMDR), 42–43
  group interventions, 48–49
  light therapy, 46
  overview, 42
  safety cues, 49–53
  somatic experiencing (SE), 42
  sound therapy, 46–47
  trauma-informed yoga, 43
polyvagal-informed interventions, healthcare
  acute risk and crisis, 58–59
  polyvagal promotions protocol, 54
  stress-management, 93–96
polyvagal-informed interventions, stakeholder management
  case study, 122–123
  clinical data incorporation, 123
  marketing tactics, 124
  target clientele, 122
Porges, Stephen, 7–8, 28
posttraumatic stress disorder (PTSD), 76
Posttraumatic Stress Disorder (PTSD) scale, 105
primary stress interventions, 94–95
Project Oxygen, 90
projection bias, 63
prosody, 47
protection state (ANS), 66
psychological construct, definition, 104
Purpose in Life Scale, 106

racial prejudice, 68–69
Regulating Resources Map, 36–37

Safe and Sound Protocol (SSP), 47
safety
  autonomic nervous system (ANS), 5
  clinical measurement, 101
  neuroception, 9
  polyvagal theory, 5
  polyvagal theory enhancements, 17
  Porges on, 7–8
safety and healthcare environment
  ANS attunement, 110
  case study, 111
  cues, 110
  lighting, 111–112
  temperature, 110
  ventilation, 110–111
safety cues (PVT)
  body language, 50
  case study, 52–53
  demeanor, 52
  eye contact, 50
  facial expressions, 50–51
  language of design, 52
  physical proximity, 51–52
  tone of voice, 50
secondary stress interventions, 95
"seeing" others skill, 92
selective attention, 63
self-regulation skills (PVT), 37–39
servant leadership style
  case study, 88
  characteristics, 87
  definition, 86–87
  pros and cons, 87–88
  ventral vagal state alignment, 87
situational leadership style
  case study, 86
  characteristics, 85
  innovative nature of, 84–85
  key principals of, 85
  pros and cons, 85–86
  requirements for, 85
skills for high-stress environment
  group meetings, 92–93
  "moments between" awareness, 92
  personal containment, 92
  "seeing" others, 92
  tactile orientation, 92
  transitional movement, 92
social brain network, 90
social engagement system
  awareness exercises, 21–23
  illustration, 9, 11
socialization state. *see* ventral vagal state

Somatic and Psychological
  Health Report
  (SPHERE), 105
somatic experiencing (SE),
  31, 42
somatic psychology
  definition, 16
  need for assessment
    development in, 107
  as paradigm departure from
    cognitive psychology,
    30–31
sound therapy
  acoustic comfort, 47
  autonomic sound
    response, 46
  definition, 46
  music of the voice, 47
  Safe and Sound Protocol
    (SSP), 47, 59
stakeholder management,
  healthcare
  collaboration case study,
    122
  healthcare providers, 121
  internal and external
    classification, 119–120
  learning research
    institutions, 121–122
  polyvagal-informed
    interventions, 122–123
  private payors, 120–121
  public payors, 120
  relevance understanding
    steps, 119
stakeholders, healthcare
  definition, 118
  example, 118–119
standardized psychological
  assessment measurement
  health scales and measures,
    105–107
  instruments, 105
  pros and cons, 105
statistical discrimination,
  63
steadfast leadership
  case study, 90
  definition, 88
  importance of, 97
  intuition and, 89

rational and nonrational
  balance, 88–89
stress and trauma
  environments, healthcare
  distress reactions, 76–77
  exposure effects, 76
  health risk behaviors,
    77–78
  leadership in, 79–80
  polyvagal theory and, 16–17
  psychiatric disorders, 77
  PTSD, 76
  responses to, 77
stress-management
  interventions, categories
  case study, 96
  primary interventions,
    94–95
  secondary interventions, 95
  summary, 93–94
  tertiary interventions, 95
stress-management
  interventions, importance
  of, 93, 96
subjective measures, healthcare
  outcomes
  case study, 103
  emotional well-being metric,
    102–103
  pros and cons, 103
sympathetic nervous
  system (SNS)
  overview, 28
  schematic of, 10
sympathetic state
  challenge activities, 57
  challenge comments,
    55–56
  change activities, 57
  change comments, 55
  definition, 13
  employment candidates, 67
  exercises, 23–25
  polyvagal ladder, 14
  stay activities, 56
  stay comments, 54

tactile orientation skills, 92
taste-based discrimination, 63
tertiary stress interventions, 95
thermal discomfort, 110

tone of voice, 50
transactional leadership
  classification
  active management by
    exception, 81
  passive management by
    exception, 81
transactional leadership style
  case study, 82
  definition, 80
  pros and cons, 81–82
  research on, 81
  rewards and
    punishments, 81
  traits, 80–81
transformational leadership
  style
  case study, 84
  characteristics, 83
  as opposite of transactional
    style, 83
  pros and cons, 83–84
  ventral vagal state
    alignment, 83
transitional movement
  awareness skill, 92
trauma-informed yoga, 43

vagus nerve, 6
ventral vagal complex (VVC)
  location and function, 8
  overview, 28
  stimulation exercises, 23
ventral vagal state
  awareness exercises, 21–23
  change comments, 59
  definition, 13
  employment candidates, 67
  polyvagal ladder, 13–14
  servant leadership style, 87
  stay activities, 56
  stay comments, 54, 59
  transformational leadership
    style alignment, 83
visual appeal, workplace design
  case study, 116
  color, 114–115
  decorations, 116
  layout, 114
  lighting, 113–114
  signage, 116

Made in the USA
Monee, IL
03 May 2026

49437981R00079